FOURTH EDITION

DEVELOPING CLINICAL PROFICIENCY

in

ATHLETIC TRAINING

FOURTH EDITION

DEVELOPING CLINICAL PROFICIENCY

in

ATHLETIC TRAINING

A Modular Approach

ATHLETIC TRAINING EDUCATION SERIES

Kenneth L. Knight, PhD, AT, FACSM, FNATA
Brigham Young University

Kirk Brumels, PhD, AT
Hope College

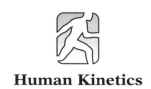

Human Kinetics

Library of Congress Cataloging-in-Publication Data

Knight, Kenneth L.
    Developing clinical proficiency in athletic training : a modular
approach / Kenneth L. Knight, Kirk Brumels. -- 4th ed.
        p. ; cm. -- (Athletic training education series)
    Rev. ed. of : Assessing clinical proficiencies in athletic training.
3rd ed. c2001.
    Includes bibliographical references.
    ISBN-13: 978-0-7360-8361-4 (soft cover)
    ISBN-10: 0-7360-8361-8 (soft cover)
    1. Physical education and training--Safety measures--Study and
teaching (Higher) 2. Sports injuries. I. Brumels, Kirk, 1966-   II.
Knight, Kenneth L. Assessing clinical proficiencies in athletic
training. III. Title. IV. Series: Athletic training education series.
    [DNLM: 1. Sports Medicine--education. 2. Athletic Injuries. 3.
Competency-Based Education--methods. QT 261 K69d 2010]
    GV344.K57 2010
    617.102'7--dc22

                                                    2009021664

ISBN-10: 0-7360-8361-8
ISBN-13: 978-0-7360-8361-4

This book is a revised edition of *Assessing Clinical Proficiencies in Athletic Training: A Modular Approach, Third Edition*, published in 2001 by Human Kinetics Publishers, Inc.

Acquisitions Editor: Loarn D. Roberston, PhD; **Series Developmental Editor:** Amanda S. Ewing; **Managing Editor:** Melissa J. Zavala; **Assistant Editor:** Christine Bryant Cohen; **Copyeditor:** Alisha Jeddeloh; **Permission Manager:** Dalene Reeder; **Graphic Designer:** Bob Reuther; **Graphic Artist:** Kathleen Boudreau-Fuoss; **Cover Designer:** Keith Blomberg; **Photographer (cover):** © Neil Bernstein; **Printer:** Versa Press

Printed in the United States of America   10   9   8   7   6   5   4   3   2

The paper in this book is certified under a sustainable forestry program.

Human Kinetics
Web site: www.HumanKinetics.com

United States: Human Kinetics
P.O. Box 5076, Champaign, IL 61825-5076
800-747-4457
e-mail: humank@hkusa.com

Canada: Human Kinetics
475 Devonshire Road Unit 100, Windsor, ON N8Y 2L5
800-465-7301 (in Canada only)
e-mail: info@hkcanada.com

Europe: Human Kinetics
107 Bradford Road, Stanningley, Leeds LS28 6AT, United Kingdom
+44 (0) 113 255 5665
e-mail: hk@hkeurope.com

Australia: Human Kinetics
57A Price Avenue, Lower Mitcham, South Australia 5062
08 8372 0999
e-mail: info@hkaustralia.com

New Zealand: Human Kinetics
P.O. Box 80, Torrens Park, South Australia 5062
0800 222 062
e-mail: info@hknewzealand.com

                                                                    E4837

CONTENTS

Foreword **ix** ■ Introduction to the Athletic Training Education Series **xi**
Preface **xv**

CHAPTER 1 **Philosophy and Principles
of Clinical Skill Development** 1

By Design or by Chaos 1
Directed Progressive Proficiency Development 2
Integrated Curriculum 2
Athletic Training Education Venues 2
Teaching Versus Learning 3
Clinical Education Is Not Clinical Experience or Work 3
Clinical Skills Versus Clinical Decision Making 3
Role of the Clinical Instructor 4
Peer Teaching for Deeper Learning 5
References 6

CHAPTER 2 **Module Program Overview** 7

Flexibility in the Program and Individual Modules 7
Modular Approach 8
Module Completion 9
Assessing Student Competency 9
Self-Paced Progress 9
Customizing for Flexibility 9
Oral and Practical Examinations 11

LEVEL 1 **Introduction to AT Clinical Education** 13

1.1 Directed Clinical Experience (Clinic Orientation and Student Staff) .. 15
   X1 Athletic Training Observation 16
   X2 Athletic Training Clinic Student Staff 17
   X3 Athletic Training Clinic Student Staff 18
1.2 Developing Clinical Skills 19
   A1 Philosophy and Principles of Clinical Education 20
   A2 Becoming a Critically Thinking Clinician 22
   A3 Foundational Behaviors of Professional Practice 1 23
1.3 Athletic Training Clinic Operations 24
   B1 Administrative Policies and Procedures 25
   B2 Injury Record Keeping 26
   B3 Athletic Training Supplies 28
   B4 Athletic Training Clinic Equipment—Small 29
   B5 Athletic Training Clinic Equipment—Major 30
   B6 Basic Health Care Nomenclature 31

1.4 Emergency and Acute Care of Injuries and Illnesses **33**
C1 Emergency and Acute Care Philosophy 34
C2 Principles of Initial Assessment 35
C3 Emergency Action Plans 36
C4 Cardiopulmonary Resuscitation 37
C5 Choking, Hemorrhaging, and Shock 38
C6 Emergency Transportation 39
C7 Medical Services (Health Center, Hospitals, Physicians) 40
C8 Rest, Ice, Compression, Elevation, and Support (RICES) 41
C9 Open Wounds 43
C10 Universal Precautions Against Bloodborne Pathogens,
    Hepatitis, and Tuberculosis 45
C11 Environmental Injury and Illness 47
C12 Anaphylaxis and Asthma Attacks 48
C13 Poison Control Center 49

1.5 O/P1 O/P Examination 1 . . . . **50**

LEVEL 2   **Individual Athletic Training Skills Development** **51**

2.1 Directed Clinical Experience (Athletic Training Staff) **53**
X4 Foundational Behaviors of Professional Practice 2 54
X5 Football Team Experience 55
X6 Basketball Team Experience 57
X7 Men's Team Sport Experience 59
X8 Women's Team Sport Experience 61
X9 Men's Individual Sport Experience 63
X10 Women's Individual Sport Experience 65
X11 High School Experience 67
X12 Sports Medicine Clinic or Industrial Experience 68

2.2 Peer Teaching and Supervision **69**
T1 Teaching Level 1 Athletic Training Students 70

2.3 Surgical Procedures **72**
D1 Basic Surgical Procedures 73
D2 Surgical Observation 74

2.4 The Body **75**
E1 Body Systems and Development 76
E2 Injury and Illness Pathology 77
E3 Exercise and Disease 78
E4 Body's Response to Injury 80

2.5 Taping, Wrapping, Bracing, and Padding **81**
F1 Ankle Taping, Wrapping, and Bracing 85
F2 Knee Taping, Wrapping, and Bracing 86
F3 Thigh and Lower-Leg Taping, Wrapping, and Padding 88
F4 Foot Care, Taping, Wrapping, and Padding 90
F5 Hip and Abdomen Taping, Wrapping, and Bracing 92
F6 Shoulder Taping, Wrapping, and Bracing 93
F7 Elbow-to-Wrist Taping, Wrapping, and Bracing 95
F8 Hand and Finger Taping and Wrapping 97
F9 Head and Neck Padding and Bracing 99

2.6 Risk Management **100**
G1 Anthropometric Measurements and Screening Procedures 101
G2 Protective Equipment Fitting 102
G3 Ergonomics and Injury Prevention 103
G4 Fitness Testing 104
G5 Flexibility Training 105
G6 Strength Training 107

2.7 Basic Nutrition, Pharmacology, and Wellness **109**
H1 Medication Resources 110
H2 Medication Physiology 111

H3 Medication Policies and Procedures. 112
H4 Basic Performance Nutrition and Supplementation. 113
H5 Eating Disorders. 115
H6 Health and Wellness 116

2.8 General Assessment and Evaluation 118
I1 Orthopedic Injury Assessment Principles 119
I2 General Medical Assessment 121
I3 Postural Assessment. 123
I4 Neurological Assessment 124
I5 Palpation 125
I6 Range-of-Motion and Strength Assessment. 126
I7 Physical Performance Measurements 128
I8 Orthopedic Injury Assessment 130

2.9 Specific Injury Assessment and Diagnosis 131
J1 Foot Injury Assessment and Diagnosis 132
J2 Ankle Injury Assessment and Diagnosis 137
J3 Lower-Leg Injury Assessment and Diagnosis. 140
J4 Knee Injury Assessment and Diagnosis. 144
J5 Thigh, Hip, and Pelvic Injury Assessment and Diagnosis 151
J6 Thorax and Lumbar Spine Injury Assessment and Diagnosis. 158
J7 Thorax and Abdominal Injury Assessment and Diagnosis 163
J8 Shoulder Injury Assessment and Diagnosis. 167
J9 Arm and Elbow Injury Assessment and Diagnosis. 173
J10 Wrist and Hand Injury Assessment and Diagnosis 178
J11 Cervical Spine Injury Assessment and Diagnosis 184
J12 Head and Facial Injury Assessment and Diagnosis. 188

2.10 General Medical Conditions, Disorders, and Diseases. 194
K1 Assessment, Diagnosis, and Care of Simple Dermatological Conditions 195
K2 Common Syndromes and Diseases. 198
K3 Common Viral and Respiratory Tract Conditions and Disorders. 200
K4 Common Cardiovascular and Gastrointestinal Tract Conditions and Disorders . 202
K5 Common Genitourinary, Gynecological, and Sexually Related Conditions,
Disorders, and Diseases 204
K6 Sudden Illnesses and Communicable Diseases 207

2.11 Therapeutic Modalities 209
L1 Therapeutic Modality Foundation 210
L2 Whirlpool. 212
L3 Moist Hot Packs 213
L4 Paraffin Bath 214
L5 Cryotherapy 215
L6 Cryokinetics 217
L7 Cryostretch 218
L8 Lymphedema Devices. 219
L9 Ultrasound 220
L10 Pulsed Shortwave Diathermy. 222
L11 Electrical Stimulation 223
L12 Therapeutic Massage. 225
L13 Traction. 227

2.12 Therapeutic Exercise. 229
M1 Range-of-Motion and Flexibility Exercises 230
M2 Joint Mobilization 232
M3 Isometric Resistance Exercises 234
M4 Isotonic Strength Training Devices 235
M5 Daily Adjustable Progressive Resistive Exercise 237
M6 Isokinetic Dynamometers 239
M7 Muscular Endurance 240
M8 Aquatic Therapy. 242
M9 Neuromuscular Control and Coordination Exercises 244
M10 Muscular Speed Exercises 246
M11 Agility Exercises. 247
M12 Plyometrics 249

M13 Cardiorespiratory Endurance 251
M14 Activity-Specific Skills 253
M15 Exercise for the Young and Old 255

2.13 O/P2 O/P Examination 2 257

LEVEL 3 **Integrating and Polishing Skills 259**

3.1 Directed Clinical Experience (Athletic Training Staff) 260
X13 Foundational Behaviors of Professional Practice 3 261
X14 Comprehensive Team Experience 262
X15 Clinical Capstone Experience 263
X16 Athletic Team Travel 264

3.2 Peer Teaching and Supervision 266
T2 Teaching and Supervising Level 2 Students 267
T3 Administering O/P Examination 1 269
T4 Teaching and Supervising Level 3 Students 270
T5 Administering Comprehensive O/P Examination 272
T6 Writing O/P Questions 273
T7 Updating Reference Material 274

3.3 Integrated Injury Management 275
N1 Musculoskeletal Assessment and Diagnosis 276
N2 General Medical Assessment and Diagnosis 277
N3 Emergency and Acute Care 278
N4 Rehabilitation Overview 279
N5 Rehabilitation Adherence and Motivation Techniques 281
N6 Rehabilitation Planning and Supervision 282

3.4 Health Care Administration 284
O1 Program Policies and Procedures 285
O2 Human Resources and Personnel Management 287
O3 Facility Management 288
O4 Fiscal Management 290
O5 Information and Data Management 291
O6 Preparticipation Medical and Physical Examination 293

3.5 Psychosocial Interactions 294
P1 Health Care Communication 295
P2 Substance Abuse 297
P3 Psychosocial Intervention 299

3.6 Professional Development 301
Q1 Regulation of Athletic Training Practice 302
Q2 Athletic Training in the Community 304
Q3 National Athletic Trainers' Association 306
Q4 Athletic Training Research 307
Q5 Educational Aids and Professional Presentation 309
Q6 Presenting Yourself to the Job Market 310

3.7 O/P3 O/P Examination 3 311

Appendix A Information for Customizing Modules 313

Appendix B Reprint of *Hyposkillia and Critical Thinking* 315

Appendix C O/P Examination 319

Appendix D NATA Competencies Embedded in Modules 323

Appendix E Master Module Completion File 329

About the Authors   **333**

FOREWORD

The changes in the fourth edition of *Developing Clinical Proficiency in Athletic Training: A Modular Approach* parallel the growth and development of our clinical teaching. Ken Knight and Kirk Brumels continue to calm the clinical education chaos and carve a structured path through the revised and expanded athletic training educational competencies. With the concept of "learning over time" still embedded in the customizable modules, this edition places increased emphasis on the roles and responsibilities of the classroom and laboratory instructors, ACIs, and students in the clinical learning *process*.

The ultimate goal of clinical education is for the student to gain mastery of the subject matter. The applications of the cognitive and psychomotor competencies are packaged together as clinical proficiencies to form a set of clinical outcomes. In other words, performing the skill only measures psychomotor competence. The proficiency measures the student's ability to integrate individual psychomotor skills into a larger objective (e.g., demonstrating the ability to identify when and when not to include the Lachman's test into a knee examination), interpreting the results, and making sound clinical judgments. Although this text is primarily based on the Athletic Training Educational Competencies, the authors have expanded certain sections to include material that are vital for skill development.

This edition places more emphasis on clinical experiences and clinical education, with the overriding theme being the professional socialization of athletic training students. The key to this text is still practice-based education, but there is an added emphasis of controlled autonomy. Students may be placed in critical thinking (i.e., decision-making positions), while patient safety is assured by an ACI or CI who only intervenes if the student does not choose the best course of action based on the situation. The socialization aspect is reinforced by a new module, Foundational Behaviors of Professional Practice, which is repeated in all 3 levels.

Three groups of modules have been added. In addition to the clarification of clinical education and clinical experience, the authors have included base modules addressing the body's systems, injury and illness pathology, exercise and disease, and the body's response to injury. These modules provide a solid foundation for building proficiency in clinical diagnosis, treatment, and rehabilitation areas. Other new additions include the much needed Professional Development section that addresses regulation of AT, the NATA, the need for (and consumption of) professional research, and the AT's role in the community.

Dr. Knight, now ably assisted by Dr. Brumels, continues to provide order to what once was the chaos of clinical education.

Chad Starkey, PhD, LAT
Associate Professor, Ohio University

INTRODUCTION TO THE ATHLETIC TRAINING EDUCATION SERIES

The six titles of the Athletic Training Education Series—*Core Concepts in Athletic Training, Examination of Musculoskeletal Injuries, Therapeutic Exercise for Musculoskeletal Injuries, Therapeutic Modalities for Musculoskeletal Injuries, Management Strategies in Athletic Training,* and *Developing Clinical Proficiency in Athletic Training*—are textbooks for athletic training students and references for practicing certified athletic trainers. Other allied health care professionals, such as physical therapists, physician's assistants, and occupational therapists, will also find these texts to be invaluable resources in the prevention, examination, treatment, and rehabilitation of injuries to physically active people.

The rapidly evolving profession of athletic training necessitates a continual updating of the educational resources available to educators, students, and practitioners. The authors of the six new editions in the series have made key improvements and have added information based on the fourth edition of the NATA Athletic Training Educational Competencies.

- *Core Concepts in Athletic Training,* which replaces *Introduction to Athletic Training,* is suitable for introductory athletic training courses. Part I of the text introduces students to mechanisms of injury, pathophysiology, and injury assessment. It also includes a chapter with some of the injuries and tests that students should be aware of. Part II introduces topics in injury examination, and part III considers the use of modalities and exercise in the therapeutic rehabilitation process. Part IV covers prevention topics such as conditioning, nutrition, protective gear, and taping and bracing. Part V introduces the managerial and legal issues relevant to clinical practice in athletic training.
- In *Examination of Musculoskeletal Injuries,* new information about sensitivity and specific- ity strengthens the evidence-based selection of special tests, and an increased emphasis on clinical decision making and problem solving and the integration of skill application in the end-of-chapter activities are now included.
- Two new chapters have been added to *Therapeutic Exercise for Musculoskeletal Injuries.* Chapter 16 focuses on arthroplasty, and chapter 17 contains information regarding various age considerations in rehabilitation. This text also provides more support of evidence-based care resulting from a blend of research results and the author's 40 years of experience as a clinician.
- The new edition of *Developing Clinical Proficiency in Athletic Training* contains 27 new modules, and embedded within it are all the 2006 NATA Athletic Training Educational Competencies. The concepts of progressive clinical skill development, clinical supervision and autonomy, and clinical decision making are introduced and explained. The nature of critical thinking and why it is essential to clinical practice are also discussed.
- The third edition of *Therapeutic Modalities for Musculoskeletal Injuries* continues to provide readers with information on evidence-based practice and includes recent developments in the areas of inflammation and laser therapy.
- The fourth edition of *Management Strategies in Athletic Training* continues to help undergraduate and graduate students master entry level concepts related to administration in athletic training. Each of the ten chapters has been thoroughly updated, with new material added on such topics as evidence-based medicine, professionalism in athletic training, health care financial management, cultural competence, injury surveillance systems, legal updates, athletic trainer compensation, and more.

The Athletic Training Education Series offers a coordinated approach to the process of preparing students for the Board of Certification examination. If you are a student of athletic training, you must master the material in each of the content areas delineated in the NATA Athletic Training Educational Competencies. The Athletic Training Education Series addresses each of the competencies sequentially while avoiding unnecessary duplication.

The series covers the educational content areas developed by the Education Council of the National Athletic Trainers' Association for accredited curriculum development. The content areas and the texts that address each content area are as follows:

- Risk management and injury prevention (*Core Concepts* and *Management Strategies*)
- Pathology of injury and illnesses (*Core Concepts, Examination, Therapeutic Exercise,* and *Therapeutic Modalities*)
- Orthopedic assessment and diagnosis (*Examination* and *Therapeutic Exercise*)
- Acute care (*Core Concepts, Examination,* and *Management Strategies*)
- Pharmacology (*Therapeutic Modalities*)
- Conditioning and rehabilitative exercise (*Therapeutic Exercise*)
- Therapeutic modalities (*Therapeutic Modalities*)
- Medical conditions and disabilities (*Examination*)
- Nutritional aspects of injury and illness (*Core Concepts*)
- Psychosocial intervention and referral (*Therapeutic Modalities* and *Therapeutic Exercise*)
- Administration (*Management Strategies*)
- Professional development and responsibilities (*Core Concepts* and *Management Strategies*)

The authors for this series—Craig Denegar, Peggy Houglum, Richard Ray, Jeff Konin, Ethan Saliba, Susan Saliba, Sandra Shultz, Ken Knight, Kirk Brumels, and I—are certified athletic trainers with well over three centuries of collective experience as clinicians, educators, and leaders in the athletic training profession. The clinical experience of the authors spans virtually every setting in which athletic trainers practice: high schools, sports medicine clinics, universities, professional sports, hospitals, and industrial settings. The professional positions of the authors include undergraduate and graduate curriculum director, head athletic trainer, professor, clinic director, and researcher. The authors have chaired or served on the NATA's most prominent committees, including Professional Education Committee, Education Task Force, Education Council, Research Committee of the Research and Education Foundation, Journal Committee, Appropriate Medical Coverage for Intercollegiate Athletics Task Force, and Continuing Education Committee.

This series is the most progressive collection of texts and instructional materials currently available to athletic training students and educators. Several elements are present in most of the books in the series:

- Chapter objectives and summaries are tied to one another so that students will know and achieve their learning goals.
- Chapter-opening scenarios illustrate the relevance of the chapter content.
- Thorough reference lists allow for further reading and research.

To enhance instruction, various ancillaries are included:

- All of the texts (except for *Developing Clinical Proficiency in Athletic Training*) include instructor guides and test banks.
- *Therapeutic Exercise for Musculoskeletal Injuries* includes a presentation package plus image bank.
- *Core Concepts in Athletic Training, Therapeutic Modalities for Musculoskeletal Injuries,* and *Examination of Musculoskeletal Injuries* all include image banks.
- *Examination of Musculoskeletal Injuries* includes an online student resource.

Presentation packages include text slides plus select images from the text. Image banks include most of the figures, tables, and content photos from the book. Presentation packages and image banks are delivered via PowerPoint, and instructors can use these to enhance lectures and demonstration sessions. Other features vary from book to book, depending on the subject matter; but all include various aids for assimilation and review of information, extensive illustrations, and material to help students apply the facts in the text to real-world situations.

The order in which the books should be used is determined by the philosophy of each curriculum director. In any case, each book can stand alone so that a curriculum director does not need to revamp an entire curriculum in order to use one or more parts of the series.

When I entered the profession of athletic training over 30 years ago, one text—*Prevention and Care of Athletic Injuries* by Klafs and Arnheim—covered nearly all the subject matter required for passing the Board of Certification examination and practicing as an entry-level athletic trainer. Since that time we have witnessed an amazing expansion of the information and skills one must master in order to practice athletic training, along with an equally impressive growth of practice settings in which athletic trainers work. You will find these updated editions of the Athletic Training Education Series textbooks to be invaluable resources as you prepare for a career as a certified athletic trainer, and you will find them to be useful references in your professional practice.

David H. Perrin, PhD, ATC
Series Editor

PREFACE

The fourth edition of *Developing Clinical Proficiency in Athletic Training: A Modular Approach* refines the pioneering approach to organizing and assessing clinical education. It continues the tradition established by earlier editions of guiding students and clinical instructors on a pathway through the maze of educational competencies required of entry-level ATs. Unchanged is the basic philosophy that students' clinical experiences must have structure, that learning clinical skills by osmosis or by just putting in time on the job is haphazard and ineffective, and that the traditional hit-and-miss system whereby students spend a specific number of hours in the athletic training clinic developing their clinical skills results in too many misses.

This new edition contains 27 new modules, and embedded within the text are all the 2006 National Athletic Trainers' Association (NATA) *Athletic Training Educational Competencies.* Some of the new modules were necessary because of new educational competencies, others were included to better cover competencies from the previous edition of this manual, and still others were stimulated by dialogue with educators and leaders while serving on the NATA Education Council Executive Committee.

What's New?

The most significant change is the addition of Dr. Kirk Brumels of Hope College as a coauthor. Kirk is a veteran clinician and clinical educator who has used the modular system for many years. But that is only the beginning; we have made many more changes that make this text a much more dynamic tool for guiding clinical skill acquisition. Following are the highlights of the changes:

- We have changed the title to *Developing Clinical Proficiency in Athletic Training: A Modular Approach* because we feel this more fully encompasses the scope of the text. While assessing clinical skills is important, there are many instruments for assessing skills. The more important role of this text is to guide students through the 1,200 educational competencies. It organizes the clinical education experience in such

a way that students progressively develop skills and competence. As a student progresses through the modules, the modules increase in complexity and integrate educational competencies from more diverse content areas. The task of clinical education is much larger than learning and passing off a list of skills. The emphasis must be on developing clinical proficiency, on putting things together. We intentionally use the singular form of proficiency to emphasize our integrated approach. Although we deal with developing proficiencies in several areas of AT, doing so gives one proficiency in the field of athletic training.

- We have added introductory material aimed at helping students and faculty better understand the integrated nature of athletic training education and how classroom, clinical skill laboratories, and clinical experiences should work together during students' education.

- The concepts of progressive clinical skill development, clinical supervision and autonomy, and clinical decision making are introduced and explained.

- The nature of critical thinking and why it is essential to clinical practice is discussed. We also give some easily understood examples of how students can enhance their critical thinking and encourage students to adopt habits of critical thinking.

- The grouping of modules has changed from four levels to three by shifting the modules from level 3 of the previous edition into levels 2 and 3. We believe this gives educators greater flexibility in adapting the program to specific curriculums. But more importantly, it has a pedagogical function by conveying the integrated and progressive nature of clinical skill development. The new titles of the levels also reflect this: Level 1: Introduction to Athletic Training Clinical Education, Level 2: Individual Athletic Training Skills Development, and Level 3: Integrating and Polishing Skills.

- In addition to the lettered listings of module groups found in previous editions, each module group has been assigned a number referencing its location and purpose within the clinical education progression.

- A new module, Foundational Behaviors of Professional Practice, has been inserted into all three levels of modules and clinical experiences. During the rewriting of the 2006 Athletic Training Educational Competencies, the Professional Education Committee of the NATA Education Council correctly surmised that the affective competencies of previous editions represented behaviors that were difficult to measure but nonetheless were essential elements of student learning and professional practice. Furthermore, these foundational behaviors permeate every aspect of professional practice and should be incorporated into every part of students' education. Inserting them into each level of skill development ensures that students and clinical instructors will have an ongoing dialogue concerning these behaviors, and it will help students adopt and develop these concepts and behaviors.

■ We have added a new element to most modules, a list of the specific NATA educational competencies embedded in the module. A table in appendix D also cross-references the competencies by listing the competency first and the modules in which that competency is embedded. We say *most modules* have this feature because some modules go beyond the NATA educational competencies with material we feel is essential to skill development. The clinical experience modules are examples.

■ There are three new groups of modules, one in each of the three levels.

– In level 1, we have added Developing Clinical Skills, a group of three modules aimed at helping students understand the difference between clinical experience and clinical education. Students are to be supervised and instructed rather than just assigned to cover the clinic and athletic practices and games. A second aim is to help develop critical thinking, by engaging students in reading, thinking about, and discussing the importance of and how to think critically. A third aim of this section is to help students take responsibility for their personal clinical skill development, thus shifting the emphasis from teaching to learning.

– The Body is a set of four new level 2 modules. These include concepts that are necessary prerequisites for subsequent modules as well as information that does not fit into other module groups. These modules are Body Systems and Development, Injury and Illness Pathology, Exercise and Disease, and Body's Response to Injury.

– Four new professional development modules are included in level 3: Regulation of Athletic Training Practice, The National Athletic Trainers' Association, the Athletic Trainer in the Community, and Athletic Training Research.

■ 16 new modules are scattered through the text as needed to enhance the existing modules. A few are combined or renamed.

■ There has also been some minor rearranging of modules in various sections.

■ As in past new editions, the prefixes (lettered listing of module groups) have changed. Again, we apologize to those who currently are using the program for the confusion that will exist during the transition into the new book. For those who are just adopting the program, the changes will make no difference. New competencies dictated additional modules and groups of modules that could not be stacked at the end of the former modules. We hope the new and updated modules will compensate for the slight confusion.

■ We have removed most references from the modules. The vast majority of students will use the texts from their didactic courses as reference material, so the listing of additional texts is irrelevant. References were important in previous editions because they were written for both curriculum and internship students. Many internship students did not have specific classes and thus needed guidance as to where to find material for the modules. The elimination of this route to certification has eliminated this need. Also, the listing of page numbers for these reference texts became obsolete with new editions of the texts.

What Is Not New?

The basic philosophy of the text, which was innovative in 1990, has now become mainstream. The debate that raged for 15 years over how many hours students should work in order to develop sufficient skills has been forgotten. The profession agrees that developing competencies is more important than putting in hours and hoping to learn by osmosis.

The purpose of this text is not to teach these skills, because there are many excellent texts that do so. Instead, its purpose is to organize these skills into a system that will help students develop the skills progressively and that will provide a systematic means of assessing that learning.

The modular approach is still intact, and appropriately it remains the subtitle of the book. Some may choose to regroup the modules so that the program more closely fits with their curriculum. Regardless of how the modules are grouped, educators and clinical instructors can be assured that by systematically working through these modules, students will develop and demonstrate all the basic clinical skills required of entry-level ATs, at least in a laboratory setting.

We continue to strongly support the peer-teaching concept contained herein, although the program can easily be used without peer teachers if an institution chooses to do so. But requiring more advanced students to work with newer students will reinforce the more advanced students' knowledge and skill mastery and will decrease the cycling or stuff-and-purge approach to learning.

Structured Clinical Experience

For years, educators have debated the most effective ways of teaching the knowledge and skills necessary to be successful professionals. Much effort, time, and money have been spent in identifying the knowledge, psychomotor skills, and attitudes of professionals. As a result, we can tell our students what knowledge, psychomotor skills, and attitudes they must master to pass the certification examination and successfully work in the field.

After many years of experience and thousands of examinations, the NATA Board of Certification (now Board of Certification, or BOC) determined that athletic training skills and knowledge cannot be learned as thoroughly with on-the-job training as with a structured curriculum. Dr. Chad Starkey, a former member of the BOC and first chair of the NATA Education Council, stated that one of the greatest needs in athletic training education is structured clinical experiences. We agree and offer a program in line with the 2006 NATA Athletic Training Educational Competencies in this new edition of *Developing Clinical Proficiency in Athletic Training: A Modular Approach.*

Philosophy and Principles of Clinical Skill Development

A thletic training students must acquire practical skills. These skills require a knowledge base, but abstract knowledge is not enough—it must be applied. Skills necessary for competent sport injury management are developed only through clinical experience. The organization of the clinical experience, however, determines the depth and breadth of a student's skill development.

The Athletic Training Educational Competencies of the National Athletic Trainers' Association specify the knowledge, skills, and clinical proficiencies necessary for an entry-level athletic trainer (AT). These competencies are organized into 12 content areas. While such an organization is necessary to ensure completeness, it gives no direction for student acquisition of knowledge and skills. This text helps educators and students organize clinical skill acquisition so as to facilitate the process. It organizes the clinical education experience in such a way that students progressively develop skills and competence. As a student progresses through the modules, the modules increase in complexity and integrate educational competencies from more diverse content areas. The task of clinical education is much larger than learning and passing off a list of skills. The emphasis must be on developing clinical proficiency and on putting things together. The aim of this program is to do just that.

By Design or by Chaos

Traditionally, the underlying assumption of clinical education in athletic training, and in most other medical fields, has been learning by osmosis—that is, if you spend enough time on the job, you will develop clinical skills by reacting to the situations you are exposed to. However, that approach is too haphazard. Students are not all exposed to the same injuries during their clinical experiences, and therefore they do not have equal opportunities to develop clinical skills. Some sports entail many more injuries than others, and within a particular sport, the number and kinds of injuries vary from week to week and from year to year. Thus, learning from actual injuries seems to be a matter of luck.

Another problem is that students often waste time during team practices. Typically, there is a rush of activity immediately before practice as athletes are taped, bandaged, and cared for in preparation for the practice, and there is also much to do after practice. But unless an athlete is injured during the practice, many students spend practice time waiting for something to happen. If students are properly directed, they can use this time to develop and refine skills.

As a result of these challenges, a plan was developed to ensure that all students can develop and demonstrate their competence in clinical skills that are basic to the athletic training profession, regardless of whether they are exposed to the situations requiring those skills during their clinical experiences. The result of these efforts is the modular program described in this book. The key is ensuring that each student is properly directed. The modular program does this by lending structure and objectivity to the process of developing clinical skills. Athletic training educators and students can be assured that those who have completed the program will have had at least laboratory experience in dealing with the most common athletic injuries. Thus, the program eliminates the hit-or-miss approach to clinical education.

A principle is a basic idea or rule that explains how something works. Function follows form, meaning behavior follows, or grows out of, basic beliefs or principles. Since the beginning of time, philosophers have suggested that people change actions by changing thinking. Students and educators should understand the following principles and be reminded of them often. Doing so will enhance students' development of clinical skills, clinical decision making, and clinical actions.

Directed Progressive Proficiency Development

The goal of AT education is to prepare competent and confident ATs prepared to assist patients to return to a pain-free active life. The goal of clinical education is to assist students to operationalize their didactic knowledge so they can correctly determine patient needs and properly intervene so as to restore or improve patients' health. To achieve these goals, clinical education must be more than spending a specified number of hours in the clinic and checking off a list of educational competencies.

Like a successful road trip, successful clinical education requires a destination or goal and a road map or detailed plan for getting there. Granted, if your goal is just to wander aimlessly, then it doesn't matter how, or to where, you wander. But developing competent clinicians requires more than aimless wandering. The concepts and principles of this chapter will help students and educators understand the importance of a structured clinical education program and how this modular approach facilitates clinical proficiency.

Integrated Curriculum

A curriculum defines a student's educational experiences. For an accredited athletic training curriculum,

these experiences are delineated by the National Athletic Trainers' Association (NATA) Athletic Training Educational Competencies and the philosophy and requirements of individual institutions (such as general education). Thus, the information that is to be taught is relatively easy. But just as important is the order in which these competencies are presented. Students should be led through their educational experiences so that they develop foundational knowledge first and then build knowledge on the foundation. This program is developed to do just that.

A second concern is that skill development should be an outgrowth of theory classes. In other words, skill development should be integrated with the presentation of theory in the classroom. Stated another way, students' clinical experiences should be a laboratory for their theory classes. Two problems arise if skill development and theory are not integrated. First, students may have to develop clinical skills without adequate background, or the application of theory may not be apparent. Second, students may get the idea that there are two programs, one involving theory classes and another involving clinical experiences wherein the student develops clinical skills as an apprentice to the athletic training clinical staff.

The sequence of modules presented in this text may not parallel the didactic class schedule in all institutions. Therefore, either the didactic class scheduling or the sequence of modules should be adjusted (as outlined in the next section) so that the curriculum is integrated.

Athletic Training Education Venues

Athletic training education occurs in three general venues, each with unique goals and objectives: didactic (classroom), clinical skills (psychomotor skills development on uninjured peers), and clinical education (psychomotor skills refinement and clinical decision making on injured patients).

Athletic training education is typically thought of as didactic (classroom) and clinical education. But clinical skills are developed in two venues: in laboratories, often called *clinical education classes,* and in the athletic training clinic with patients. Both are necessary, but the approach and the outcomes are different.

Clinical education, by definition, occurs with patients (1). Although important, classes or laboratories where clinical skills are taught, practiced, and tested are not clinical education; they are clinical skills classes. Calling both clinical skills classes and patient interaction *clinical education* conveys the idea that they are the same and therefore one can substitute for the other, but such is not the case. Assessing a classmate's knee is not the same as assessing a patient who hobbled in because of extreme knee pain. An uninjured peer does not give the same feedback after having a thumb taped as does an athlete who must grip a sporting implement with that hand.

Both clinical skills classes and clinical education have pros and cons. Clinical skills classes cannot duplicate patient experience, but they do allow students to refine psychomotor and clinical decision-making skills before laying hands on a patient. They allow the budding clinician to rehearse clinical skills: to solidify the questions to be asked, develop a systematic pattern of palpation, practice proper positioning of both clinician and patient, and practice applying pressure to the body part in the proper direction and with the correct amount of pressure. Similar to most mental and psychomotor skills in life, it takes repetition and even failure to become proficient. The adage "Prior practice prevents poor performance" is true for students.

As important as clinical skills classes are, however, they are no substitute for clinical experiences. Clinical decision making can only develop from mentored patient care. Clinical skills classes serve only to prepare a student for clinical education at the bedside of patients.

Some minimize the importance of didactic classes, claiming that classroom education is more valuable in passing the Board of Certification (BOC) exam but that clinical education is more important in preparing for real life as an AT (2). Neither function exists in a vacuum, however. They are interrelated, and they feed off each other in a properly designed curriculum.

Athletic training practice involves surveying a situation, determining patient needs, and then pursuing a course of action that will meet those needs. An adequate knowledge base is necessary to establish needs and determine appropriate action. The greater the knowledge base, the greater the possibility that the clinical decision will lead to quicker and completer resolution of the problem. All other things being the same, the more effective the classroom instruction is, the better the clinical decision making will be and the better the health care for the patient. However, all the knowledge in the world is valueless if it cannot be applied. As stated earlier, athletic training is the application of knowledge, so without good clinical education, much of the value of the classroom education is wasted.

Teaching Versus Learning

Classroom and clinical educators, program directors, and educational administrators and leaders should always remember that first and foremost, it's all about student learning (3). A teacher's efforts are of no use if the student does not learn. This does not mean that teachers should pander to students; however, putting the student first also means setting high expectations for them and correcting them with kindness when necessary.

In addition, students, with guidance from faculty, must take responsibility for their skill development. The clinical curriculum should be organized so that students become proficient in the psychomotor competencies in a sequential manner. Students should have monthly, weekly, and even daily clinical education goals. They should suggest the agenda for instruction by demonstrating clinical skills to their clinical instructor. They should approach their clinical instructor with the attitude of "will you help me perform the Lachman test?" rather than "what are you going to teach me today?" As stated previously, the clinical instructor's role is to assist students, not direct their clinical education.

Clinical Education Is Not Clinical Experience or Work

Experience and work are not necessarily education. Students' time in the clinic traditionally has been referred to as *clinical experience* or *working in the clinic*. Indeed, students do work and provide much service to the athletic department or clinic to which they are assigned, but calling this time *work* or *experience* suggests that the students are there to put in time, learning whatever they pick up along the way. Calling this experience *clinical education* reminds all that the primary purpose is to develop clinical skills and clinical decision making.

Clinical Skills Versus Clinical Decision Making

Clinical skills and clinical decision making are not the same. Clinical skills are the performance of clinical activities. Clinical decision making is determining which clinical activity to engage in during a specific situation and interpreting the results of the activity. Clinical skills can range from performing a simple diagnostic test that is relatively easy to interpret, such as an ankle drawer test, to performing a complex activity, such as evaluating the ankle of a patient with unknown pathology. Clinical skills are easier to develop than clinical decision making. Both must be emphasized.

Skill Development Must Be Integrated

Clinical skills require background knowledge, practice on uninjured people, and application to patients. In other words, skill development requires didactic knowledge, which generally comes from lecture classes, followed by practice in a clinical skills class and then application during clinical experience. These educational activities should be integrated (4), occurring in temporal proximity. Clinical skills classes should be organized so that students are practicing skills related to the knowledge they are studying in their didactic classes. Once they become minimally proficient with the skills, they should be directed to opportunities to apply those skills to patients during their clinical experiences. Too often, students complete these three aspects of their education in isolation. It seems that many students complete a clinical internship independent of classes. Students' proficiency will be greatly enhanced if these three educational experiences are integrated.

Progression by Design

Clinical skill development and decision making occur by design and must be progressive (4). Complex skills are developed only after a proper foundation of knowledge and basic and moderate skills is established. A weak person who wants to lift 100 lb (45 kg) cannot do so by immediately lifting 100 lb. He must begin by lifting 10 lb (4.5 kg) and then progress incrementally up to 100 lb. Curriculums must be designed so that students begin by developing basic skills and making simple decisions, incrementally progressing to complex skills and decisions.

Role of the Clinical Instructor

Clinical education requires clinical instructors, practitioners, or clinicians who are actively caring for patients. Although their educational role is essential, it is secondary to their clinical role of treating patients (1, 5). This means they should not be expected to develop lesson plans for what they teach, nor will their delivery be systematic. They teach to the moment, meaning they will share insights concerning patient care as they are

caring for the patient or in response to student questions. Inquisitive students will get much more from their clinical experiences than those who sit back and wait for their clinical instructor to "teach them."

Avoid the phrase *educators versus clinicians,* which many use to differentiate between those who hold academic positions and those who hold staff positions. Although these two groups of professionals have different educational roles and responsibilities, both are critical to student education. The phrase implies that clinicians are not educators. This is both false and degrading, and it dishonors the essential role that clinicians play in student education. If there is a need to differentiate between these two groups, use the terms *academics* and *clinicians.* Academics are those who hold academic positions at a college or university and clinicians are those who hold clinical or staff positions. But regardless of how human resources classifies ATs, if they are teaching students, they are educators.

Clinician First

Clinical instructors are clinicians first. Students and academics must realize that clinical instructors' first priority is patient care. They are interested in helping students learn, but not at the expense of their main job. Clinical instructors should not be expected to develop lesson plans or to determine what the students' educational needs are each day. They are a resource, not a curriculum director (see the next principle).

Autonomy and Direct Supervision

Autonomy can and must occur during direct supervision. Many in the profession believe that autonomy can only occur in the absence of supervision, that direct supervision prevents students from acting autonomously. It is true that in the absence of supervision, students are forced to rely on their own resources, to make independent decisions, and to innovate when necessary. But this behavior can also take place in the presence of supervision if clinical instructors and students plan for it, discuss it, and make it part of the clinical experience.

Clinical supervision ranges from hovering over students to make sure they do everything correctly to quietly observing the situation and then answering questions and suggesting alternatives after students have independently handled the situation. Many great clinical instructors have mastered the art of evaluating injuries through the hands of a student. They stand back physically but are fully invested mentally in the evaluation process. They watch the evaluation carefully, noting the patient's response to the student's intervention. They may suggest at times that the student perform this or that test in addition to what has already been done. Allowing such autonomy does not compromise patient care if the student has been properly prepared for the situation and if the instructor is attentive in spite of being silent.

Intervention by the clinical instructor during either skill performance or clinical decision making should be great with beginning students and progressively decrease with time until it is minimal with advanced students. Autonomy is a matter of attitude, not proximity.

Appropriate Student Assignments

Students should be appropriately assigned to clinical instructors. Too often students are assigned to a clinical instructor with little regard for the students' skill development needs. Clinical instructors are often assigned students with little experience one rotation and students with advanced skills the next. This is OK if the clinical instructor has different responsibilities during the year, but not if the clinical instructor's duties are fairly homogeneous. Failing to take into consideration students' previous experience can create confusion concerning what to expect from the students, how to integrate the students with the clinical instructor's daily activities, and the amount of autonomy to allow the students. Too often this results in an internship experience where skill development is haphazard.

There must be a differentiation between the clinical responsibilities of a first-semester student and a last-semester student. These responsibilities must be planned in advance of the assignment and some thought must go into what types of students are assigned to specific clinical instructors at various times of the year. For example, a clinical instructor will have different responsibilities for the team she is assigned to during the competitive season than during the off-season.

Daily Interaction and Feedback

Students and clinical instructors need daily interaction and feedback. Clinical activity is not passive. It is not the students shadowing the clinical instructor, nor is it students acting as independent caregivers. The student must be actively engaged in caring for patients and making clinical decisions which are followed by discussion and feedback by the clinical instructor. Dialogue should occur multiple times daily between students and clinical instructors. This daily feedback should concern skills, clinical decision making, and the foundational behaviors of professional practice.

Seize the Moment

Teaching moments are powerful. Organizing clinical experiences so that students develop skills and decision making in a sequential manner should not negate the power of teaching moments. Even though a specific situation may be beyond the level of the student, when a great teaching moment arises, the educator should seize it. Some students may not get as much from the experience as they would later in their educational career, but the specific situation may not occur again. Teaching moments should not be passed up. Such experiences often remain with the student for a lifetime.

Peer Teaching for Deeper Learning

Another unique aspect of this approach is that it incorporates peer teaching. Peer teachers are more experienced students. Level 1 students look to level 2 students as peer teachers, and level 2 students look to level 3 students as peer teachers. A student can be a peer teacher to someone who is less advanced and receive peer teaching by someone who is more advanced. Although this concept was rejected by some athletic training educators when it was introduced in the first edition of this text, there is growing evidence that it is an effective pedagogical tool (6, 7, 8, 9). The program can be used without peer teachers if an institution so desires; we have attempted to make the program very flexible.

The peer teacher's role is to help less advanced students by demonstrating, encouraging, and correcting newer students as they practice skills. Peer teachers assist after the clinical skills and the background information are taught by faculty or clinical instructors and before the student demonstrates proficiency to an ACI.

Peer teaching benefits both the student as well as the peer teacher. An old educational adage states, "The best way to learn something is to teach it." In medicine, the philosophy is stated as "See it, do it, teach it." In working with younger students, peer teachers deepen their own understanding of and ability to apply the material. Thus, although students will demonstrate a beginning mastery of skills, their understanding will deepen as they teach the skills to others. Such an approach helps them to learn over time; they can't just pass off a competency, forget it, and then move on to the next one.

A potential hazard of peer teaching is that if students are not conscientious when they serve as peer teachers, they may teach skills inadequately or may fail to correct mistakes. Over time learning could deteriorate. This can be prevented by careful supervision by clinical instructors and by a systematic program of oral and practical examination of all students. Such a program, as the one outlined in this text, helps students keep abreast of what they have learned and thus helps them be better peer teachers. Above all, remember that peer teaching is part of mastering the skill and is not the final approval that the student has mastered the skill.

References

1. Knight, KL. Educational Perceptions vs. Reality; Classroom and Clinical Education. *Athletic Training Education Journal.* 2006;1(Apr-Dec):15-17.

2. Huggins, R. Student Corner: Classroom vs. Clinic: Where Should Students Focus Their Learning? *NATA News*, Sept. 2006.

3. Knight, KL. It's All About Students . . . Learning *Athletic Training Education Journal.* 2007;2(Jan-Mar):3.

4. Knight, KL. Progressive Skill Development and Progressive Clinical Experience Responsibility. *Athletic Training Education Journal.* 2008;1(Jan-Mar):2-4.

5. Brumels, K., Beach, A. Role Orientation of Certified Athletic Trainers at Institutions of Higher Education. *Athletic Training Education Journal.* 2008;1(Jan-Mar):5-12.

6. Henning, JM., Weidner, TG., Jones, J. Peer-assisted learning in the athletic training clinical setting. *J Athl Train.* 2006 (Jan-Mar);41(1):102-8.

7. Weidner, TG., Popp, JK. Peer-assisted learning and orthopaedic evaluation psychomotor skills. *J Athl Train.* 2007 (Jan-Mar);42(1):113-9.

8. Secomb, J. A systematic review of peer teaching and learning in clinical education. *J Clin Nurs.* 2008 Mar;17(6):703-16.

9. Loke, AJ, Chow, FL. Learning partnership--the experience of peer tutoring among nursing students: a qualitative study. *Int J Nurs Stud.* 2007 Feb;44(2):237-44.

Module Program Overview

The modular approach consists of 148 modules organized into three levels and 20 groups. Each module contains instructions to the student for demonstrating specific knowledge, developing specific skills, practicing the skills on a peer, practicing the skills on a patient, and then demonstrating competence to a peer teacher and to an ACI. All the NATA 2006 *Athletic Training Educational Competencies* required for entry-level ATs are embedded within the modules.

Modules are arranged into three levels (numbered) and subgrouped within those levels (alphabetized and numbered), partly based on the difficulty and complexity of the skills involved. Students begin developing simple skills and progressively acquire more complex ones. Basic skills developed during many level 1 and 2 modules are later integrated into more complex skills required for level 3 modules.

Flexibility in the Program and Individual Modules

There is great variety among athletic training curriculums. Although all should teach the minimum knowledge and psychomotor skills required by the NATA education competencies, the manner in which this material is organized into a 4- or 5-year course of study differs from one institution to another. Thus, the way this modular program is adapted to individual

institutions will vary. Much flexibility is built into the program, and with a bit of foresight and planning, the program can be adapted to most situations.

For example, most universities want their students to learn taping and bandaging skills before modality application. Thus, taping and bandaging are grouped together as F modules (level 2.5), and therapeutic modality application is presented within a group of L modules (level 2.11). Institutions that require students to master modality application before taping may simply tell students to complete the L group of modules before the F group. One institution has redefined the levels; it has some F, some L, and some M modules together in its level 2.1. Individual institutions may also elect to add or eliminate modules to meet their needs and specific philosophies. As stated previously, skill development should be parallel to theory classes, so modules should parallel theory classes.

In addition to program flexibility, there also must be individual module flexibility. Most modules are generic, applying to students from any school. Others, such as those that deal with filling out clinic records and becoming familiar with local hospitals and physicians' offices, will be specific to each institution. Procedures have been incorporated that allow specific modules to be customized for each institution (see pages 9 and 313).

In addition to ensuring that students encounter a variety of injuries and situations, the modular program provides guidelines for assigning students to specific responsibilities commensurate with their skill development. Thus, students need not worry about being in over their heads, and the athletic training staff can be confident that students are able to perform assigned duties. More importantly, it facilitates increased clinical responsibility which requires increasingly complex clinical decision making and thus enhances student growth, development, and proficiency.

Modular Approach

The structured but flexible program presented in this text is designed to guide students through experiences that will help them develop the skills and background necessary to be a competent entry-level AT. The program will assist them in applying the knowledge gained in didactic classes.

Module Program

The program consists of 150 modules arranged into three levels and 20 blocks of related subject matter. Most of these blocks (A-Q) are located within a specific level; however, blocks X, T, and O/P are found across the three levels Each subject area (block) is designated by a letter:

- Modules A through Q develop specific clinical skills.
- X modules involve directed clinical experience.
- T modules are peer-teaching modules.
- O/P modules are oral and practical examinations.

The following sections will give an idea of the three levels of experience as well as the format of the modules, the subject matter of each block of modules, and the number of modules in each block.

Level 1: Introduction to AT Clinical Education

3 X modules: Directed Clinical Experience (Clinic Orientation and Student Staff)

3 A modules: Developing Clinical Skills

6 B modules: Athletic Training Clinic Operations

13 C modules: Emergency and Acute Care of Injuries and Illnesses

1 O/P module: O/P Examination 1

Level 2: Individual Athletic Training Skills Development

9 X modules: Directed Clinical Experience (Athletic Training Staff)

1 T module: Peer Teaching and Supervision

2 D modules: Surgical Procedures

4 E modules: The Body

9 F modules: Taping, Wrapping, Bracing, and Padding

6 G modules: Risk Management

6 H modules: Basic Nutrition, Pharmacology, and Wellness

8 I modules: General Assessment and Evaluation

12 J modules: Specific Injury Assessment and Diagnosis

6 K modules: General Medical Conditions, Disorders, and Diseases

13 L modules: Therapeutic Modalities

15 M modules: Therapeutic Exercise

1 O/P module: O/P Examination 2

Level 3: Integrating and Polishing Skills

4 X modules: Directed Clinical Experience (Athletic Training Staff)

6 T modules: Peer Teaching and Supervision

6 N modules: Integrated Injury Management

6 O modules: Health Care Administration

3 P modules: Psychosocial Interactions

6 Q modules: Professional Development

1 O/P module: O/P Examination 3

Module Format

Each module consists of four parts:

1. Objective or purpose of the module
2. NATA educational competencies that are embedded within the module
3. List of competencies, or specific performance skills that students must master to reach the objective
4. Proficiency demonstration and space for signatures of didactic, skills, peer, and clinical teachers when students have demonstrated that they are proficient in performing the competencies

Overlap in Modules

The modules have some overlap (for example, with the modules for anatomy in the ankle and lower leg). Modules were developed as self-contained units, so it is reasonable that some overlap would occur. Rather than looking at this as extra work, look at it as an opportunity to solidify the material.

Module Completion

Students work on modules within a block (i.e., modules designated by the same letter) simultaneously and complete them in any order. In general, they should complete all modules within each block before moving to the next block of modules. Three exceptions are the F, T, and X modules; these are designed to be completed at the same time as other blocks within the same level.

Assessing Student Competency

The skills included in the modules are skills students will use for a lifetime. Therefore, students should not cycle knowledge here (i.e., memorize, pass a test, forget the material, and move on to the next module of material). The knowledge base of the skill should be taught in one or more classes. Clinical education is the time to solidify that knowledge and apply it. Students should review the material, work with peer teachers, and then practice, study, and practice. When they can use the material confidently, they pass it off, first to a peer teacher and then to an ACI.

Most work on the modules (both developing the skills and demonstrating competence) should occur during regular athletic training clinical hours as students study with each other during slack times. Work on modules must not interfere with clinical duties, but there usually is a great deal of time to work on them during team meetings, practices, and so on.

Self-Paced Progress

The program allows students to work at their own pace. However, there are a minimum and a maximum number of modules that should be completed each semester. Timing is also important, for two reasons. First, it is not fair for peer teachers to have many students come to them at the end of the semester wanting to pass off numerous modules. For most students, the end of the semester is a busy time. Second, our experience is that students sacrifice quality when they try to pass off many modules at once.

To force the issue of proper timing, we encourage the policy of allowing students to pass off any number of modules during the first part of the semester, one or two modules per week during the last half of the semester, and none during the last week or final exams. This prevents students from putting off module completion.

When Do Students Work on Modules?

Students generally will demonstrate mastery of module competencies during clinical skills classes and during their clinical education assignments. They should make arrangements ahead of time with an appropriate module supervisor (professor or clinical instructor), allowing extra time in case an emergency arises that would require the student's or supervisor's services in caring for athletes. Before the conference with a module supervisor, students should have an intellectual understanding of the purpose and knowledge required for the module, practice the skills of the module, practice testing, and then practice demonstrating all module skills to a peer.

Role of Module Supervisors

Module supervisors must be approved clinical instructors (ACI) and are responsible for the instruction and final approval of each student's competency at completing individual modules. Module supervisors may use various methods for module content instruction including athletic training faculty and fellow students at the college or university. Students may supervise and initiate peer instruction for module work at a level they have completed; however, an ACI must evaluate the clinical competency or proficiency prior to independent practice. For example, a person at level 3 can supervise people working on levels 1 and 2. The last section of each module provides space for module supervisors to sign off on students' proficiency demonstrations.

Customizing for Flexibility

There are three ways to customize this program to institutional needs and preferences, and none of these ways is the right way. The organization of the complete curriculum, the needs of the athletic department for athletic training services, the types of equipment available, and the skills and techniques used by the full-time athletic training staff all affect the clinical education program. Most of these differences can be addressed by customizing the information in modules, adding and subtracting modules, customizing the levels and blocks of modules, and customizing the module rotation.

Customizing Modules

Most modules deal with standard or generic information and apply to all clinical settings. Others, however, involve specific details that vary from one institution to another and therefore will need to be customized. For instance, module A2 pertains to record keeping. Because most universities use their own forms, students need to become familiar with the forms and record-keeping system of their program.

The following modules require customization:

■ B2 Injury Record Keeping: Records and forms used in the athletic training clinics, such as daily treatment logs, individual treatment sheets, insurance forms, and referral to physician

■ B3 Athletic Training Supplies: Selected medical supplies used during this module to acquaint students with the types of supplies used in the athletic training clinic and with how they are inventoried, purchased, stored, and made accessible for daily use

■ B4 Athletic Training Clinic Equipment—Small: Selected medical equipment used during this module to acquaint students with the types of small equipment (e.g., braces, pads) used in the athletic training clinic and with how the items are inventoried, purchased, stored, and made accessible for daily use

■ B5 Athletic Training Clinic Equipment—Major: Equipment used during this module to familiarize students with the major equipment used in the athletic training clinic (such as ice machines and therapeutic modalities) and with how the items are purchased

■ C7 Medical Services (Health Centers, Hospitals, Physicians): Names of community medical services to which students may need to transport patients, such as physicians' offices, hospital emergency rooms, and hospital outpatient surgical units

■ M4 Isotonic Strength Training Devices: Weight training equipment that students use in clinics for rehabilitation, including at least one piece of equipment for each major joint of the body

Skipping or Adding Modules

Some modules in this book may not apply to an athletic training program, and there may be additional modules that the curriculum director or head AT has written for the program. Obtain these from the curriculum director or head AT.

Customizing Module Levels and Blocks

Institutional philosophy and how theory classes are organized and taught will dictate differences in the order of developing clinical skills. The order and grouping of modules may be customized to fit the institutional philosophy.

Customizing Module Rotation

Institutions with clinical education phases ranging from 2 to 4 years have adopted this program. Table 2.1 shows possible schedules for work on the three levels within clinical education sequences of various lengths; certainly there are other possibilities.

Recognizing Customized Modules

The athletic training curriculum director or head AT will provide the appropriate information for the modules listed. This information may include one or more of the lists supplied in appendix A or may be specific to the situation. Get the needed information from the athletic training curriculum director or head AT.

Creating a Customized Reference Library

Students will rely on the texts, notes, and assigned readings from their didactic classes for most of the background knowledge needed to complete modules. But there are many other excellent references for this material. Each program should maintain a library of

TABLE 2.1 Possible Schedules for Progression Through the Clinical Proficiency Levels

	COMPETENCY LEVEL		
Program length (yrs)	1	2	3
2-1/2	1st semester	2nd-3rd semesters	4th-5th semesters
3	1st semester	2nd-4th semesters	5th-6th semesters
3-1/2	1st semester	2nd-5th semesters	6th-7th semesters
4	1st-2nd semesters	3rd-6th semesters	7th-8th semesters

these additional references in a place convenient to the major athletic training clinic where students will complete most of their clinical education. Students and faculty will add to this library as they collect additional references.

Following are examples of references used by Oregon State University for its module on bloodborne pathogens:

- 1995 NATA position statement on bloodborne pathogens
- Oregon Occupational Health and Safety Administration (OSHA) bloodborne pathogens regulations
- American Liver Foundation lay summaries on hepatitis A, B, and C
- June 1996 Oregon State University safety bulletin on tuberculosis and infection control in the workplace

Oral and Practical Examinations

Oral and practical (O/P) examinations are an excellent way of helping students develop clinical skills. Comprehensive O/P examinations should be given at key points in the program to assess students' retention of the skills they have learned up to that point in the program. In addition, short O/P exams every 3 to 4 weeks help students keep up to date on material they have mastered. Thus, O/P exams are an additional way of helping students learn over time. Obviously, students don't have to review the skills they use more often in the clinic, but skills that they do not use regularly will be lost without regular review and repetition.

Incorporating O/P exams in the curriculum offers other benefits as well. First, the exams help students with their peer teaching. By keeping current with their newly developed skills, students have a stronger knowledge base from which to teach. A second benefit of O/P exams is that they help students perform under pressure, which often is a part of real-life situations when athletes are injured during crucial athletic con-

tests. A third benefit is that O/P exams help prepare students psychologically for the NATA Board of Certification (BOC) examination.

We have found success in organizing short O/P exams as follows. Miniexams are given every 3 weeks during the weekly practicum class. Students are divided into groups of five, all within the same level. Each group is given three copies of five O/P questions. The students draw lots to determine their order: Number 1 is the examinee, 2 is the model, and 3, 4, and 5 are the examiners. The examiners then administer the first exam. After the first exam is completed, the students change positions, the second exam is given, and so on until all five group members have been examined. In less than an hour, all students can be tested at their own level. Clinical instructors rotate from group to group to monitor the exams.

Three comprehensive O/P exams are built into this program—one after each level. More could be given, but there should be at least three. The important thing is that the exams are comprehensive and students know they must prepare for them. These exams can be administered by faculty or peers; we have done both for more than 20 years and find benefits to both methods. We organize O/P exams on a single day, with each student scheduled for a 30- to 40-minute exam and multiple exams occurring in different rooms. When we use peer examiners, faculty or ACIs administer the first few exams, and students rotate into the examiner role after they have been tested themselves. Typically they are involved in five exams: one as the examinee, one as the model, and three as an examiner. When the exams are administered by peers, always have an ACI closely monitor the examination sites.

Students find that giving exams is also an important learning experience. They frequently recognize aspects of the skill they may have forgotten. And when peers forget critical aspects of a skill that they were able to perform in a group study session the previous night, students also see firsthand the effects of pressure on performance and the need for constant repetition.

Appendix C contains the instructions and a sample O/P question.

Introduction to AT Clinical Education

The goal of clinical education is to allow students to operationalize their didactic knowledge and apply the clinical skills learned in the classroom and clinical skills courses on actual patients. The modules of this text are organized to help students progress from simple skills to complex, integrated skills. Level 1 modules are divided into four groups:

1. Directed Clinical Experience
2. Developing Clinical Skills
3. Athletic Training Clinic Operations
4. Emergency and Acute Care of Injuries and Illnesses

The directed clinical experience modules allow students to observe the structure, operation, and practice of athletic training and thus understand more completely the practice of athletic training in various settings. Observation, interviews, and writing a case study are tangible opportunities for students to experience the profession directly.

Modules for developing clinical skills require students to examine their responsibility in the development of clinical skills. Athletic training education consists of didactic (classroom) and clinical (hands-on) learning. Knowledge and basic skills should be taught in classroom and laboratory settings, whereas clinical education is the process of developing these clinical skills during patient care. For this process to be effective, students must understand that they are to be actively involved in creating opportunities for clinical instruction and clinical practice. The modules in this section ask the student to reflect on and examine behaviors associated with self-directed learning and professional practice of health care providers in general and ATs specifically.

The modules for athletic training clinic operations provide a directed introduction to the operation of athletic training clinics in general and specifically the locations where students will be obtaining their clinical experiences. Working on these modules will help students understand what an athletic training clinic is, how it operates, and how it interfaces with the larger world of athletic heath care.

Finally, students will begin to obtain skills needed for acute care of injuries and illnesses. Competency in emergency and acute care of injuries and illness is a vital component of health care. Improper emergency care can create a cascade of negative events, potentially leading to

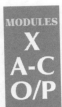

MODULES

X

A-C

O/P

permanent physical disabilities and even death. On the other hand, appropriate initial care is the basis for effective medical treatment, creating an optimal environment for best-case scenarios and timely recovery. Therefore, it is vital that students demonstrate proficiency in basic emergency and acute care of athletic injuries; these skills are paramount to additional psychomotor skills relating to the field of athletic training.

Note: The term *clinic* used herein refers to any facility where athletic health care is administered. A clinic is a center for physical examination and treatment of patients who are able to move about and are not hospitalized. Most athletic departments call the place where ATs perform their labors a *training room* even though it often is a suite of rooms and there is little training going on. We believe that *athletic injury clinic, sports medicine clinic,* or *athletic health clinic* more appropriately describe what goes on in a clinic. It is an allied health care facility and should be referred to as such. We will use the term *athletic training clinic* in this text, which contains elements of the past yet recognizes that the facility is a health care facility.

Level 1 includes 26 modules, organized into five groups:

1. 3 X modules—Directed Clinical Experience (Clinic Orientation and Student Staff) . . 15
2. 3 A modules—Developing Clinical Skills 19
3. 6 B modules—Athletic Training Clinic Operations 24
4. 13 C modules—Emergency and Acute Care of Injuries and Illnesses 33
5. 1 O/P module—O/P Examination 1 50

Directed Clinical Experience (Clinic Orientation and Student Staff)

Experience is one of life's greatest teachers. The impact of each experience depends on the background knowledge the student has gained from previous experiences. The debate over which type of education is best for students is often concluded with the understanding that a combination of both learning styles is most effective. The purpose of this book is to facilitate an organized process of obtaining clinical experiences that will help prepare students for entry-level competence.

For a long time, ATs were educated through basic classroom coursework and significant clinical experiences that focused on experiential learning. Many members of the profession were educated using this method, but it became clear that the knowledge gained was dependent upon the experiences and situations that the individual AT was exposed to. In 1995, leaders within the profession formed the Education Reform Task Force and explored the best ways and practices for athletic training education. In 1997, they released recommendations stating that education of ATs should consist of both classroom (didactic) education and clinical (experiential) education (NATA Education Task Force 1997). To have an effective clinical experience, the student first must be knowledgeable in the didactic information that forms the foundation for clinical activities and skills, which are then performed for a patient's benefit based on sound clinical decision making.

Clinical experiences blend didactic knowledge (learned in a classroom) and clinical skills (learned in a laboratory setting) to make clinical decisions for appropriate medical care of patients (Knight 2006). The experience of responding to actual patient complaints using the knowledge taught in class and the skills learned in a laboratory setting is true clinical education and serves a vital role in the development of athletic training skills. There are certain skills that cannot be taught in class or labs and must be experienced for complete synthesis.

During the course of this program, students should work closely with faculty and their clinical instructors to obtain quality clinical experiences for multiple sport and health care settings. To obtain the greatest benefit from the clinical experience, students *must* be active participants in the process. They should work closely with a clinical instructor in providing care with skills that they are competent in. Each student should take an active role in the process and apply the knowledge learned from class and lab to truly experience the clinical application.

References

Knight, K.L. 2006. Education perceptions versus reality; classroom and clinical education. *Athletic Training Education Journal* 1: 15.

NATA Education Task Force. 1997. Recommendations to reform athletic training education. *NATA News* Feb: 16-24.

Due at the end of semester

Athletic Training Observation

Objective

Become familiar with the clinical aspect of the athletic training profession.

Competencies

~~1.~~ Spend at least 30 hours observing the activities and operation of an athletic training clinic. You will be assigned specific times that you are to attend, and you may be assigned to different athletic training clinics if your school has more than one. Keep track of your time on a time sheet provided by your program director.

students

2. Interview at least two ~~staff~~ ATs and write brief reports of the interviews. Include in your reports information such as what a typical day is like for the trainers, the worst day they have had, the kind of day they hope they will never have, their best day, why they chose athletic training as a career, what they like most and dislike most about their career, what they might do differently if they could start over, and so forth.

Audrey Paige

3. In the form of a journal manuscript, write a case report of an injured athlete whom you observe during your experiences. See the author's guide of the *Journal of Athletic Training* for guidelines and tips. You can find this guide in any issue of the *Journal of Athletic Training* or on the journal Web site: www.journalofathletictraining.org. Your report should cover at least 3 weeks and contain the pertinent events and information concerning an athlete's injury, the care provided, and how this case relates to protocols given in standard athletic training texts. In each report include the following:

   a. A brief introduction in which you state why you selected the case
   b. Personal data (age, sex, race, marital status, and occupation when relevant, but not name)
   c. Chief complaint and history of present complaint (including symptoms)
   d. Results of physical examination (e.g., "Physical findings relevant to the rehabilitation program were . . .").
   e. Medical history (surgery, laboratory results, exam, and so on)
   f. Diagnosis

   g. Treatment and clinical course (immediate care and rehabilitation, including specific dates and times)
   h. Criteria for return to competition
   i. How the patient handled competition
   ✗ A discussion in which you compare this case with protocols published in standard athletic training texts

Proficiency Demonstration

APPROVED BY
(date and signature)

1. Time sheet
   ACI _____

2. Interview
   ACI _____

3. Case report
   ACI _____

COMMENTS

1. Case study - Audrey & paige

2. injury report - moe

_____

_____

_____

_____

_____

_____

Athletic Training Clinic Student Staff

Objective

Develop and polish basic clinical skills, gain experience, and develop confidence working in the clinic.

Competencies

1. Assist full-time and student staff in preventing, treating, and rehabilitating sport injuries. Continue the experience until you have completed at least half of the level 1 modules. You should confine your activities to observing techniques and clinical skills you are unsure of and performing only those skills you have passed (i.e., those that an ACI has signed off on). Thus, your activities and responsibilities will be limited to level 1 skills at the beginning of the experience and will increase as the experience progresses. You will be assigned specific times that you are to attend, and you may be assigned to different athletic training clinics if your college has more than one or has an outreach program to other local colleges or high schools.

2. Discuss your skill development progress with an ACI.

Proficiency Demonstration

Obtain the signature of an ACI when you have completed this module.

APPROVED BY
(date and signature)

1. Assisting clinic staff
   ACI _____

2. Interview
   ACI _____

COMMENTS

_____

_____

_____

_____

_____

_____

Athletic Training Clinic Student Staff

Objective

Continue to gain experience and develop confidence as you develop new clinical skills and polish those already learned.

Competencies

1. Assist full-time and student staff in preventing, treating, and rehabilitating sport injuries. Continue the experience until you have completed all level 1 modules. You should confine your activities to observing techniques and clinical skills you are unsure of and performing only those skills you have passed off (i.e., those that an ACI has signed off on). Thus, your activities and responsibilities will be limited to level 1 skills at the beginning of the experience and will increase as the experience progresses. You will be assigned specific times that you are to attend, and you may be assigned to different athletic training clinics if your college has more than one or has an outreach program to other local colleges or high schools.

2. Discuss your skill development progress with an ACI.

Proficiency Demonstration

Obtain the signature of an ACI when you have completed this module.

APPROVED BY
(date and signature)

1. Assisting clinic staff
   ACI _____

2. Interview
   ACI _____

COMMENTS

_____

_____

_____

_____

_____

_____

Developing Clinical Skills

There is an old adage, "Function follows form," and British writer James Allen stated, "Every action and feeling is preceded by a thought," and "as a man thinketh, so is he." We have found these statements to be true in our private and professional lives, and the concepts in the first two modules will help students get more out of their didactic and clinical education. By understanding the big picture (philosophy and principles), educators and students will better understand the process of developing clinical skills and clinical decision making, and therefore they will maximize their efforts.

Critical thinking is essential to becoming a critical clinician. Getting clinicians to think critically is a concern of medical and allied health educators. Simple techniques to promote critical thinking are presented in the A2 module.

The foundational behaviors of professional practice are the first of three modules that encourage students to integrate the core values of athletic training practice into their lives. According to the NATA educational competencies, these behaviors permeate professional practice and should be incorporated into every part of the educational program.

Philosophy and Principles of Clinical Education

Objective

Understand the philosophy and principles of clinical education so as to enhance your clinical skill development.

NATA Athletic Training Educational Competencies embedded in this module: none

Competencies

1. Review the NATA Athletic Training Educational Competencies and then discuss the following concepts with at least one didactic educator, one level 2 peer, and one clinical educator.

  a. What role do these competencies play in your professional development?
  b. Define and differentiate among cognitive competencies, psychomotor competencies, and clinical proficiencies.
  c. Discuss the meaning of *proficient* and *mastery* as applied to these competencies.
  d. Where is this required educational content taught in your athletic training education program?

2. Read chapters 1 and 2 of this text and then discuss the following concepts with at least one didactic educator, one level 2 peer, and one clinical educator.

  a. Purpose of clinical education
  b. Clinical education versus clinical experience
  c. Education versus work
  d. Critical thinking
  e. Clinical decision making
  f. Student ownership of clinical education

Proficiency Demonstration

1. Develop appropriate subject knowledge through coursework (C), verbal conversation (V), quizzes (Q), worksheets (W), or other approved activities (O).

2. Practice and reinforce the skills in clinical skills and laboratory courses.

3. Refine your skills by observing peer teachers and clinical instructors as they perform the skills (preferably on patients), discussing the competencies with peer teachers and clinical instructors, practicing alone and with others, and then demonstrating proficiency to a peer teacher.

4. Demonstrate your proficiency to an ACI.

APPROVED BY
(date and signature, and mode for didactic)

1. Role of clinical competencies

Didactic _____

Peer _____

ACI _____

2. Competency typology

Didactic _____

Peer _____

ACI _____

3. Proficiency versus mastery

Didactic _____

Peer _____

ACI _____

4. Integration of competencies into curriculum

Didactic _____

Peer _____

ACI _____

5. Purpose of clinical education

Didactic _____

Peer _____

ACI _____

6. Clinical education versus clinical experience

Didactic _____

Peer _____

ACI _____

7. Education versus work

Didactic _____

Peer _____

ACI _____

8. Critical thinking

Didactic _____

Peer _____

ACI _____

9. Clinical decision making

Didactic _____

Peer _____

ACI _____

10. Student ownership of clinical education

Didactic _____

Peer _____

ACI _____

COMMENTS

_____

_____

_____

_____

Becoming a Critically Thinking Clinician

Objective

Develop an understanding of the need for critical thinking in athletic training practice and of some basic skills to help you become a critically thinking clinician.

NATA Athletic Training Educational Competencies embedded in this module: none

Competencies

1. Read *Hyposkillia and Critical Thinking: What's the Connection?* (see appendix B), and then write a reflective essay on your interpretation of the article and how it relates to your clinical education and eventual health care practice. Include the following points in your essay:

  a. Hyposkilliacs
  b. Critical thinking
  c. Characteristics of a critically thinking clinician

Proficiency Demonstration

1. Read the material.

2. Write a reflective essay.

3. Discuss the concepts with a professor, a peer, and a clinical instructor.

APPROVED BY
(date and signature, and mode for didactic)

1. Essay and discussion

   Didactic _____

   Peer _____

   ACI _____

COMMENTS

_____

_____

_____

_____

_____

_____

Foundational Behaviors of Professional Practice 1

Objective

Discuss how ATs should conduct themselves when acting in a professional capacity, including behavior toward others, such as patients, colleagues, coaches and athletic department staff, and the general public.

NATA Athletic Training Educational Competencies embedded in this module: None specifically; these behaviors are to be infused throughout every aspect of the educational program.

Competencies

Define and discuss the following as they relate to how you should conduct yourself as you practice athletic training.

    a. Primacy of the patient

    b. Team approach to practice

    c. Legal practice

    d. Ethical practice

    e. Knowledge advancement

    f. Cultural competence

    g. Professionalism

Proficiency Demonstration

    1. Develop appropriate subject knowledge through coursework (C), verbal conversation (V), worksheets (W), or other approved activities (O).

    2. Discuss the concepts with a professor, a peer, and a clinical instructor.

APPROVED BY
(date and signature, and mode for didactic)

  1a. Patient primacy

    Didactic _____

    Peer _____

    ACI _____

  1b. Team approach

    Didactic _____

    Peer _____

    ACI _____

  1c. Legal practice

    Didactic _____

    Peer _____

    ACI _____

  1d. Ethical practice

    Didactic _____

    Peer _____

    ACI _____

  1e. Knowledge advancement

    Didactic _____

    Peer _____

    ACI _____

  1f. Cultural competence

    Didactic _____

    Peer _____

    ACI _____

  1g. Professionalism

    Didactic _____

    Peer _____

    ACI _____

COMMENTS

_____

_____

_____

_____

_____

_____

_____

Level 1.3

Athletic Training Clinic Operations

This group of modules is designed to help students learn the policies and procedures of the athletic training department of the institution and of the primary athletic training clinics where they will be engaged in clinical education. Observing the operation of the clinics and developing familiarity with policies and procedures, record keeping, supplies, and equipment will prepare students to participate with their clinical instructors in providing health care.

Administrative Policies and Procedures

Objective

Become familiar with the responsibilities, policies, and procedures of your athletic training department.

NATA Athletic Training Educational Competencies embedded in this module: AD-C15, AD-C17, AD-C18

Competencies

1. Identify and discuss each athletic training and sports medicine facility at your school. In your discussion, include the following:

  a. Name and location of the facility
  b. Primary purpose of the facility
  c. Typical daily schedule of activities at the facility
  d. Staff assigned to the facility
  e. Safety policies (e.g., security, fire, hazards)

2. Describe the regular (daily and weekly) cleaning and maintenance responsibilities of students and staff at each facility.

3. Read the administrative policies and procedures manual of your athletic training department. Then discuss its major points with a peer and an ACI.

Proficiency Demonstration

1. Practice and reinforce these competencies by reviewing your class notes and texts, observing peer teachers and certified or licensed professionals as they perform the skills, discussing the competencies with peer teachers and professionals, practicing alone and with a peer, and then demonstrating proficiency to a peer teacher.

2. Demonstrate your proficiency to an ACI.

APPROVED BY
(date and signature)

1. Facilities
   Peer _____

   ACI _____

2. Maintenance
   Peer _____

   ACI _____

3. Policies and procedures manual
   Peer _____

   ACI _____

COMMENTS

_____

_____

_____

_____

_____

_____

Injury Record Keeping

Objective

Learn why record keeping is essential to athletic training clinic operations and how to keep such records, and demonstrate the ability to maintain records with sensitivity to patient confidentiality.

NATA Athletic Training Educational Competencies embedded in this module: AD-C2, AD-C3, AD-C9, AD-P5, AD-P6, AD-P7, DI-C17, EX-P6

Competencies

1. Discuss the importance of record keeping in the following areas:

   a. Improving patients' health care
   b. Internal communication (with patients and among staff)
   c. External communication (with coaches, administrators, physicians, family, and insurance companies)
   d. Preventing lawsuits
   e. Research

2. Discuss why patient confidentiality is a necessary part of injury record keeping, and discuss three ways of ensuring patient confidentiality.

3. Demonstrate your ability to select and use standardized record-keeping methods by comparing and contrasting the major aspects of the SOAP, HIPS, and HOPS systems of injury record keeping.

4. For each of the records (or components of a record) in the subsequent lettered list, do the following:

   – Discuss the purpose of the record.
   – Demonstrate how to fill it out using correct terminology.
   – Demonstrate how to communicate record contents verbally and in writing using correct terminology.
   – Discuss where and how long the record is filed in the short term.
   – Discuss where and how long the record is filed in the long term.
   a. Injury and illness incident reports, including assessment, diagnosis, and initial disposition and plans
   b. Rehabilitation
   c. Physician referral
   d. Insurance and billing
   e. Individual progress and release notes
   f. Coach's updates

5. Discuss the following U.S. regulations concerning responsible records management, as well as common violations of these acts that you should avoid.

   a. Health Insurance Portability and Accountability Act (HIPAA)
   b. Family Educational Rights and Privacy Act (FERPA)

6. Demonstrate the ability to organize patient files to allow systematic storage and retrieval.

7. Demonstrate the ability to enter data into the injury software program of your athletic training clinic. (If your clinic does not use injury software, obtain a brochure for a current program and describe its major features.) w/ a student

Proficiency Demonstration

1. Practice and reinforce these competencies by reviewing your class notes and texts, observing peer teachers and certified or licensed professionals as they perform the skills, discussing the competencies with peer teachers and professionals, practicing alone and with a peer, and then demonstrating proficiency to a peer teacher.

2. Demonstrate your proficiency to an ACI.

APPROVED BY
(date and signature, and mode for didactic)

1. Importance of record keeping _PM_
   Didactic _____
   Lab _____
   Peer _____
   ACI _____

2. Confidentiality _PM_
   Didactic _____
   Lab _____
   Peer _____
   ACI _____

3. Standardized methods _PM_
   Didactic _____
   Lab _____
   Peer _____
   ACI _____

4a. Injury and illness

Didactic _____

Lab _____

Peer _____

ACI _____

4b. Rehabilitation

Didactic _____

Lab _____

Peer _____

ACI _____

4c. Physician referral

Peer _____

ACI _____

4d. Insurance documentation

Didactic _____

Lab _____

Peer _____

ACI _____

4e. Individual progress notes

Didactic _____

Lab _____

Peer _____

ACI _____

4f. Coach's updates

Didactic _____

Lab _____

Peer _____

ACI _____

5. Federal regulations

Didactic _____

Lab _____

Peer _____

ACI _____

6. Record storage

Didactic _____

Lab _____

Peer _____

ACI _____

7. Computer software

Peer _____

ACI _____

COMMENTS

_____

_____

_____

_____

_____

_____

_____

Athletic Training Supplies

Objectives

Become familiar with the functions of medical supplies commonly used by ATs and how these supplies are purchased, inventoried, stored, and used at your institution.

NATA Athletic Training Educational Competencies embedded in this module: AD-C2, AD-C3, AD-C12

Competencies

1. Discuss the purpose of the medical supplies on the list supplied by your clinical supervisor. (Note: This short list of items is intended as a random sampling of your knowledge of where athletic training supplies and equipment are kept, as well as their intended function. The list is not all-inclusive.)

2. Locate one of each item from the list in competency 1 in the daily work area of your athletic training clinic and from the bulk storage area.

3. Discuss the established plan for restocking supplies in work areas (shelves and treatment areas).

4. Assist others in restocking supplies on three separate days.

5. Browse through at least two athletic training or medical supply catalogs. As you do so, identify five items in each catalog that are in your supply area and three items that are not used at your institution.

6. Explain the annual inventory process used by your athletic training department. Explain how each form is filled out.

7. Discuss how supplies are purchased by your institution, including bulk purchases and regular replacement purchases.

Proficiency Demonstration

1. Practice and reinforce these competencies by reviewing your class notes and texts, observing peer teachers and certified and licensed professionals as they perform the skills, discussing the competencies with peer teachers and professionals, practicing alone and with a peer, and then demonstrating proficiency to a peer teacher.

2. Demonstrate your proficiency to an ACI.

APPROVED BY
(date and signature)

1. Supply use *PM*
   Peer _____
   ACI _____

2. Supply stores *PM*
   Peer _____
   ACI _____

3. Restocking plan
   Peer _____
   ACI _____

4. Restocking
   Peer _____
   ACI _____

5. Catalogs *PM*
   Peer _____
   ACI _____

6. Annual inventory process
   Peer _____
   ACI _____

7. Purchasing supplies
   Peer _____
   ACI _____

COMMENTS

_____

_____

_____

_____

Athletic Training Clinic Equipment—Small

Objective

Become familiar with the function of medical equipment commonly used by ATs and how these supplies are purchased, inventoried, stored, and used at your institution.

NATA Athletic Training Educational Competencies embedded in this module: AD-C12, AC-C2, AC-C3, TM-C8

Competencies

1. Discuss the use of the medical equipment on the list supplied by your clinical supervisor. (Note: This short list of items is intended as a random sampling of your knowledge and understanding of where athletic training supplies and equipment are kept, as well as their intended function. The list is not all-inclusive.)

2. Locate one of each item from the list in competency 1 in the daily work area of your athletic training clinic or from the bulk storage area.

3. Discuss the established plan for distributing these equipment items to patients. Which items are considered disposable, and which are returned by the patient for reuse by someone else?

4. Browse through at least two athletic training or medical supply catalogs. As you do so, identify five items in each catalog that are in your supply area and three items that are not used at your institution.

Proficiency Demonstration

1. Practice and reinforce these competencies by reviewing your class notes and texts, observing peer teachers and certified and licensed professionals as they perform the skills, discussing the competencies with peer teachers and professionals, practicing alone and with a peer, and then demonstrating proficiency to a peer teacher.

2. Demonstrate your proficiency to an ACI.

APPROVED BY
(date and signature)

1. Purpose

   Peer _____

   ACI _____

2. Storage

   Peer _____

   ACI _____

3. Distribution

   Peer _____

   ACI _____

4. Catalogs

   Peer _____

   ACI _____

COMMENTS

_____

_____

_____

_____

_____

_____

Athletic Training Clinic Equipment—Major

Objective

Become familiar with the names, locations, and uses of the medical instruments and machines used to treat and rehabilitate injured athletes.

    NATA Athletic Training Educational Competencies embedded in this module: TM-C8

Competencies

1. As you stroll through your athletic training clinic, name each piece of medical equipment and explain its main purpose.

2. Browse through at least two athletic training or medical equipment catalogs. As you do so, identify two types of equipment in each catalog that are used in your athletic training clinic and two types that are not used at your institution.

Proficiency Demonstration

1. Practice and reinforce these competencies by reviewing your class notes and texts, observing peer teachers and certified and licensed professionals as they perform the skills, discussing the competencies with peer teachers and professionals, practicing alone and with a peer, and then demonstrating proficiency to a peer teacher.

2. Demonstrate your proficiency to an ACI.

APPROVED BY
(date and signature)

    1. Purpose

        Peer _____

        ACI _____

    2. Catalogs

        Peer _____

        ACI _____

COMMENTS

_____

_____

_____

_____

_____

_____

Basic Health Care Nomenclature

Objective

Develop an understanding of basic nomenclature used in both verbal and written communication within an athletic training clinic. Begin to use appropriate health care nomenclature relating to human anatomy, movement, injuries, illness, diagnosis, treatment, and rehabilitation during your daily interactions with faculty, ACI, staff, peers, and patients.

   NATA Athletic Training Educational Competencies embedded in this module: AC-C4, AC-C6, AD-P6, DI-C4, DI-C5, DI-C16, PH-C2

Competencies

   1. Using a medical or health care dictionary (e.g., Stedman's, Taber's, Mosby's) or www.onelook.com, list and define the following:
   a. 10 common medical prefixes and 10 common suffixes
   b. 10 common prescription medication terms or abbreviations
   c. 10 common medical root words pertaining to external anatomy
   d. 10 common medical root words pertaining to internal anatomy
   e. 10 common medical verbs or adjectives
   f. 15 common medical terms relating to body fluids, colors, and substances or chemicals (5 each)

   2. Using a medical or health care dictionary, textbook, or other reference source, do the following:
   a. List and define the three cardinal planes as they relate to the human body.
   b. List and define five common medical terms relating to directional movements of body parts or joints.
   c. List and define 10 common medical terms relating to musculoskeletal injury.
   d. List and define 10 common medical terms relating to systemic illness.

Proficiency Demonstration

   1. Develop appropriate subject knowledge through worksheets (W) or other approved activities (O).

   2. Practice and reinforce the skills in clinical skills and laboratory courses.

   3. Refine your skills by observing peer teachers and clinical instructors as they perform the skills (preferably on patients), discussing the competencies with peer teachers and clinical instructors, practicing alone and with others, and then demonstrating proficiency to a peer teacher.

   4. Demonstrate your proficiency to an ACI.

APPROVED BY
(date and signature, and mode for didactic)

1a. Medical prefixes and suffixes
   Didactic _____
   Lab _____
   Peer _____
   ACI _____

1b. Pharmacology nomenclature and abbreviations
   Didactic _____
   Lab _____
   Peer _____
   ACI _____

1c. External anatomy root words
   Didactic _____
   Lab _____
   Peer _____
   ACI _____

1d. Internal anatomy root words
   Didactic _____
   Lab _____
   Peer _____
   ACI _____

1e. Medical verbs and adjectives
   Didactic _____
   Lab _____
   Peer _____
   ACI _____

1f. Bodily fluids, colors, and substances and chemicals
   Didactic _____
   Lab _____
   Peer _____
   ACI _____

2a. Cardinal planes

Didactic _____

Lab _____

Peer _____

ACI _____

2b. Directional movement

Didactic _____

Lab _____

Peer _____

ACI _____

2c. Musculoskeletal injury

Didactic _____

Lab _____

Peer _____

ACI _____

2d. Systemic illness

Didactic _____

Lab _____

Peer _____

ACI _____

COMMENTS

_____

_____

_____

_____

_____

Emergency and Acute Care of Injuries and Illnesses

For many practicing ATs employed in traditional settings, the fear of catastrophic or fatal injury to patients under their care is a real concern. Though it is impossible to completely eliminate the inherent risks associated with sport and physical activity, several steps can be taken to lessen the severity of the outcomes from emergency care situations. They can be summed up as the five Ps of acute care: preparation, policy, procedure, planning, and practice. Every AT should prepare for emergency care by creating researched policies and procedures and practicing their implementation.

Preparation for emergency situations starts with having written, understood, and rehearsed policies and procedures. A good emergency action plan (EAP) is effective in managing or avoiding altogether many situations requiring emergency care. The prevention and response procedures outlined in these types of documents help eliminate much of the confusion and chaos that can surround urgent care scenarios. Proper equipment and practice also increase the chances of avoiding the cascade of negative events that surround poorly prepared emergency reactions.

The following is a list of basic emergency care situations that the AT should be prepared to respond to according to procedures outlined in an emergency action plan:

1. Cardiopulmonary resuscitation (CPR)
2. Choking, hemorrhaging, and shock
3. Emergency transportation
4. Fractures, dislocations, and other musculo-skeletal injuries
5. Referral to medical services (health center, hospital, physicians)
6. Rest, ice, compression, elevation, and support (RICES)
7. Open wounds
8. Universal precautions against bloodborne pathogens, hepatitis, and tuberculosis
9. Environmental injury and illness
10. Anaphylaxis and asthma attacks
11. Poisoning

Other acute injuries and illnesses may present themselves depending on the employment setting, and the AT must be able to recognize and respond to them with sound medical care and judgment. These modules teach and reinforce the importance of individual skills relating to acute care of injuries and illnesses. However, many emergency care situations will force the AT to combine these skills and provide more comprehensive care in response to the needs of the patient.

As will be discovered later, appropriate emergency and acute care for non-life-threatening injuries is a critical first step in the rehabilitation process. Providing proper care creates an environment that optimizes the natural recovery process. Appropriate assessment, splinting, immobilization, RICES application, and wound care minimize the risks of additional and compounding injury, control the inflammatory process, reduce secondary injuries, and set the stage for complete rehabilitation.

Emergency and Acute Care Philosophy

Objective

Develop an understanding of the initial and secondary assessment, care, and referral responsibilities for ATs providing appropriate emergency and acute care within their work setting.

NATA Athletic Training Educational Competencies embedded in this module: AC-C1, AC-C5, AC-C10, AC-C11, AC-C16, AC-C17, AC-C20, AD-C17

Competencies

1. Discuss local, state, and national legal concerns regarding the rendering of care for emergency and acute injuries and illnesses by an AT.

2. Discuss moral and ethical issues regarding the rendering of care for emergency and acute injuries and illnesses by an AT.

3. Describe the steps and purpose of the initial assessment during emergency or acute care of injuries and illnesses.

4. Describe the steps and purpose of the secondary assessment during emergency or acute care of injuries and illnesses.

5. Describe how the following actions help an AT become better prepared to provide care for acute and emergency injuries and illnesses:

    a. Understand the uses of and obtain appropriate first aid and emergency care equipment (e.g., splints, backboard, oxygen, emergency medications, bandages).

    b. Initiate or summon an emergency medical services (EMS) response.

    c. Perform diligent and persistent monitoring of acute or emergency injuries and illnesses.

    d. Understand which, when, and why certain injuries and illnesses need referral.

    e. Understand the principles of RICES (rest, ice, compression, elevation, and support) application.

Proficiency Demonstration

1. Develop appropriate subject knowledge through coursework (C), verbal conversation (V), quizzes (Q), worksheets (W), or other approved activities (O).

2. Practice and reinforce the skills in clinical skills and laboratory courses.

3. Refine your skills by observing peer teachers and clinical instructors as they perform the skills (pref-erably on patients), discussing the competencies with peer teachers and clinical instructors, practicing alone and with others, and then demonstrating proficiency to a peer teacher.

4. Demonstrate your proficiency to an ACI.

APPROVED BY
(date and signature, and mode for didactic)

1. Legal issues

    Didactic _____

    Lab _____

    Peer _____

    ACI _____

2. Moral and ethical issues

    Didactic _____

    Lab _____

    Peer _____

    ACI _____

3. Initial assessment philosophy

    Didactic _____

    Lab _____

    Peer _____

    ACI _____

4. Secondary assessment philosophy

    Didactic _____

    Lab _____

    Peer _____

    ACI _____

5. Preparation

    Didactic _____

    Lab _____

    Peer _____

    ACI _____

COMMENTS

_____

_____

Principles of Initial Assessment

Objective

Develop an understanding of the common life-threatening injuries seen in various athletic training settings. Explain the purpose of an initial assessment, as well as the emergency equipment and supplies needed to perform it.

NATA Athletic Training Educational Competencies embedded in this module: AC-C1, AC-C2, AC-C3, AC-C5, AC-C9, AC-C10, AC-C11, AC-C12, AC-P1

Competencies

1. Discuss life-threatening injuries or illnesses an AT might be exposed to that are caused by the following:

    a. Trauma
    b. Diseases
    c. Conditions
    d. Illnesses

2. Describe the purpose of the initial assessment during emergency and acute care of injuries or illnesses.

3. List and explain the purpose of the components that make up the initial assessment.

4. Discuss the first aid supplies and equipment an AT would need in various work settings.

    a. Provide rationale for inclusion or exclusion of aforementioned supplies and equipment based on individual settings and circumstances.
    b. Demonstrate understanding of care, maintenance, and calibration of equipment and supplies as necessary.
    c. Be able to locate first aid supplies and equipment in the athletic training clinics and competitive areas at your institution.

Proficiency Demonstration

1. Develop appropriate subject knowledge through coursework (C), verbal conversation (V), quizzes (Q), worksheets (W), or other approved activities (O).

2. Practice and reinforce the skills in clinical skills and laboratory courses.

3. Refine your skills by observing peer teachers and clinical instructors as they perform the skills (pref-erably on patients), discussing the competencies with peer teachers and clinical instructors, practicing alone and with others, and then demonstrating proficiency to a peer teacher.

4. Demonstrate your proficiency to an ACI.

APPROVED BY
(date and signature, and mode for didactic)

1. Life-threatening injuries and illnesses

    Didactic _____

    Lab _____

    Peer _____

    ACI _____

2. Initial assessment purpose

    Didactic _____

    Lab _____

    Peer _____

    ACI _____

3. Initial assessment components

    Didactic _____

    Lab _____

    Peer _____

    ACI _____

4. Supplies and equipment

    Didactic _____

    Lab _____

    Peer _____

    ACI _____

COMMENTS

_____

_____

_____

Emergency Action Plans

Objective

Demonstrate ability to implement an emergency action plan (EAP) for an activity, setting, or event.

NATA Athletic Training Educational Competencies embedded in this module: AC-P1, AC-P2, AC-P3, AC-P4, AD-C15, AD-C16, AD-C18

Competencies

1. Obtain a copy of an EAP from the policies and procedures manual of your athletic training department, and discuss in detail its key elements.

2. Explain triage and how you would triage in an emergency situation with numerous injuries of various degrees of seriousness.

3. Demonstrate your ability to react to an emergency:

    a. Survey the scene.
    b. Perform a primary survey to determine if a life-threatening condition exists.
    c. Simulate activation of EMS.
    d. Perform a secondary survey to determine the status of non-life-threatening conditions.
    e. Simulate management of typical non-life-threatening conditions.

4. With peers, practice management of a suspected cervical spine fracture of a football player, including removal from the field of play.

Proficiency Demonstration

1. Develop appropriate subject knowledge through coursework (C), verbal conversation (V), quizzes (Q), worksheets (W), or other approved activities (O).

2. Practice and reinforce the skills in clinical skills and laboratory courses.

3. Refine your skills by observing peer teachers and clinical instructors as they perform the skills (preferably on patients), discussing the competencies with peer teachers and clinical instructors, practicing alone and with others, and then demonstrating proficiency to a peer teacher.

4. Demonstrate your proficiency to an ACI.

APPROVED BY
(date and signature, and mode for didactic)

1. EAP
   Didactic _____
   Lab _____
   Peer _____
   ACI _____

2. Triage
   Didactic _____
   Lab _____
   Peer _____
   ACI _____

3. React and evaluate
   Didactic _____
   Lab _____
   Peer _____
   ACI _____

4. Cervical neck care
   Didactic _____
   Lab _____
   Peer _____
   ACI _____

COMMENTS

_____

_____

_____

_____

_____

Cardiopulmonary Resuscitation

Objective

Be able to perform rescue breathing and external chest compressions to prolong life.

NATA Athletic Training Educational Competencies embedded in this module: AC-C1, AC-C3, AC-C5, AC-C9, AC-C10, AC-C11, AC-C16, AC-P1, AC-P2, AC-P3, RM-C7

Competencies

1. Demonstrate your competence in cardiopulmonary resuscitation (CPR) and automated external defibrillator (AED) use by having a valid Professional Rescuer CPR and AED certification through the American Red Cross or Basic Life Support (BLS) Healthcare Provider certification through the American Heart Association.

2. Discuss how long your certification is valid, how you can become recertified, and the BOC continuing education requirement for CPR and AED.

Proficiency Demonstration

Show your current CPR and AED card.

APPROVED BY
(date and signature)

Peer _____

ACI _____

Choking, Hemorrhaging, and Shock

Objective

Develop and demonstrate the skills necessary to recognize and manage choking, severe hemorrhage, and shock.

NATA Athletic Training Educational Competencies embedded in this module: AC-C1, AC-C2, AC-C3, AC-C5, AC-C8, AC-C9, AC-C12, AC-C13, AC-C14, AC-C27, AC-P1, AC-P2, AC-P3, AC-P4

Competencies

1. Discuss choking. Explain when you would use the following and then demonstrate each:

    a. Abdominal thrust and chest compressions—standing
    b. Abdominal thrust and chest compressions—lying
    c. Abdominal thrust and chest compressions—sitting
    d. Abdominal thrust and chest compressions on people of different sizes
    e. Finger sweep

2. Discuss why severe hemorrhaging is a medical emergency and how to control it. Then demonstrate the following:

    a. Application of pressure bandage
    b. Direct pressure

3. Discuss shock, how you would treat a patient in shock, and the consequences of not properly treating such a patient.

Proficiency Demonstration

1. Develop appropriate subject knowledge through coursework (C), verbal conversation (V), quizzes (Q), worksheets (W), or other approved activities (O).

2. Practice and reinforce the skills in clinical skills and laboratory courses.

3. Refine your skills by observing peer teachers and clinical instructors as they perform the skills (preferably on patients), discussing the competencies with peer teachers and clinical instructors, practicing alone and with others, and then demonstrating proficiency to a peer teacher.

4. Demonstrate your proficiency to an ACI.

APPROVED BY
(date and signature, and mode for didactic)

1. Choking

    Didactic _____

    Lab _____

    Peer _____

    ACI _____

2. Hemorrhaging

    Didactic _____

    Lab _____

    Peer _____

    ACI _____

3. Shock

    Didactic _____

    Lab _____

    Peer _____

    ACI _____

COMMENTS

_____

_____

_____

_____

_____

_____

Emergency Transportation

Objective

Learn how to transport athletes from the field or court after injuries of various degrees of seriousness.

NATA Athletic Training Educational Competencies embedded in this module: AC-C1, AC-C2, AC-C3, AC-C6, AC-C22, AC-C23, AC-C24, AC-C25, AC-C26, AC-C30, AC-C31, AC-C32, RM-C17, RM-P5

Competencies

1. Explain the procedures for obtaining an ambulance for the following:
   a. An athlete at your university
   b. A nonathlete university student

2. Demonstrate proper care of an athlete with a suspected spinal injury, including stabilization and spine board or body splint.

3. Demonstrate transportation off the field without a stretcher (e.g., manual conveyance technique for a sprained ankle or knee).

4. Demonstrate selection and application of splints (traditional, air, or vacuum) for the following:
   a. Dislocated tibial-talar joint
   b. Fractured midhumerus
   c. Fractured distal radius
   d. Fractured femur
   e. Subluxated patella
   f. Sprained elbow

Proficiency Demonstration

1. Develop appropriate subject knowledge through coursework (C), verbal conversation (V), quizzes (Q), worksheets (W), or other approved activities (O).

2. Practice and reinforce the skills in clinical skills and laboratory courses.

3. Refine your skills by observing peer teachers and clinical instructors as they perform the skills (preferably on patients), discussing the competencies with peer teachers and clinical instructors, practicing alone and with others, and then demonstrating proficiency to a peer teacher.

4. Demonstrate your proficiency to an ACI.

APPROVED BY
(date and signature, and mode for didactic)

1. Ambulance
   Didactic _____
   Lab _____
   Peer _____
   ACI _____

2. Spinal injury
   Didactic _____
   Lab _____
   Peer _____
   ACI _____

3. Transportation without stretcher
   Didactic _____
   Lab _____
   Peer _____
   ACI _____

4. Splints
   Didactic _____
   Lab _____
   Peer _____
   ACI _____

COMMENTS

_____

_____

_____

_____

_____

Medical Services (Health Center, Hospitals, Physicians)

Objective

Become familiar with the facilities and personnel of the medical facilities you will encounter while caring for injured athletes.

NATA Athletic Training Educational Competencies embedded in this module: AD-C20, AD-C21, PD-C9

Competencies

1. Visit the ambulance service that typically provides services to your institution. Discuss the role and typical duties of emergency medical technicians (EMTs) and how you can interact with them when they are called to the institution.

2. Complete a tour of the student health center, hospital, or clinic where athletes are cared for when they need care beyond what you can administer in the athletic training clinic. Have the person conducting the tour sign in the following space. In addition, write the names and phone numbers of following health center personnel. (Note: See if any of these positions have different titles at your university. If so, write the correct title in place of the incorrect one in the following list.)

Proficiency Demonstration

1. EMT _____

Phone _____

2. Tour director _____

Phone _____

Health center director _____

Phone _____

Assistant director _____

Phone _____

Physician _____

Phone _____

Physician _____

Phone _____

Physician _____

Phone _____

Physician _____

Phone _____

Head nurse _____

Phone _____

Assistant head nurse _____

Phone _____

Pharmacist _____

Phone _____

X-ray technician _____

Phone _____

Proficiency Demonstration

Complete a tour of the previously mentioned facilities and discuss the highlights of each tour with a peer teacher and then an ACI.

APPROVED BY
(date and signature, and mode for didactic)

1. EMT and ambulance service date

Peer _____

ACI _____

2. Health care facility date

Peer _____

ACI _____

COMMENTS

_____

_____

_____

_____

_____

_____

Rest, Ice, Compression, Elevation, and Support (RICES)

Objective

Develop and demonstrate the skills necessary to provide appropriate initial care for acute sprains, strains, and contusions.

NATA Athletic Training Educational Competencies embedded in this module: AC-C17, AC-C18, AC-C33, AC-P4, RM-C18

Competencies

1. Demonstrate application of RICES for initial care of the following conditions. Indicate how long each should be applied and reapplied and criteria for removal.

 a. Sprained ankle
 b. Strained hamstring
 c. Dislocated finger
 d. Dislocated shoulder

2. Demonstrate the ability to help an athlete use crutches by properly fitting the crutches, instructing the athlete in crutch walking technique (swing and three-point gaits), coaching the athlete while practicing walking, and correcting the athlete as necessary. Tell when to use each gait and how to help an athlete progress to normal walking.

3. Demonstrate application of two sling types (one using elastic wrap) to an athlete with a shoulder injury.

 a. Elastic wrap sling
 b. Nonelastic wrap sling

Proficiency Demonstration

1. Develop appropriate subject knowledge through coursework (C), verbal conversation (V), quizzes (Q), worksheets (W), or other approved activities (O).

2. Practice and reinforce the skills in clinical skills and laboratory courses.

3. Refine your skills by observing peer teachers and clinical instructors as they perform the skills (preferably on patients), discussing the competencies with peer teachers and clinical instructors, practicing alone and with others, and then demonstrating proficiency to a peer teacher.

4. Demonstrate your proficiency to an ACI.

APPROVED BY
(date and signature, and mode for didactic)

1a. RICES—sprained ankle
 Didactic _____
 Lab _____
 Peer _____
 ACI _____

1b. RICES—strained hamstring
 Didactic _____
 Lab _____
 Peer _____
 ACI _____

1c. RICES—dislocated finger
 Didactic _____
 Lab _____
 Peer _____
 ACI _____

1d. RICES—dislocated shoulder
 Didactic _____
 Lab _____
 Peer _____
 ACI _____

2. Crutch use
 Didactic _____
 Lab _____
 Peer _____
 ACI _____

3a. Sling—elastic wrap
 Didactic _____
 Lab _____
 Peer _____
 ACI _____

3b. Sling—nonelastic wrap

Didactic _____

Lab _____

Peer _____

ACI _____

COMMENTS

_____

_____

_____

Open Wounds

Objective

Develop and demonstrate the skills necessary to provide initial care to open wounds.

NATA Athletic Training Educational Competencies embedded in this module: AC-C14, AC-C15, AC-P3, AC-P4, EX-C1, TM-C1

Competencies

1. Define and explain how the following types of open wounds occur during athletic activities:

   a. Abrasion
   b. Laceration
   c Puncture
   d. Incision
   e. Avulsion

2. For each of the wound types in competency 1, demonstrate and explain the following:

   a. Use universal precautions.
   b. Stop bleeding with direct and indirect pressure.
   c. Cleanse the wound.
   d. Disinfect the wound.
   e. Treat the wound with ointment.
   f. Dress the wound.
   g. Protect the wound during practice and competition.
   h. Manage the wound through the healing process.

3. For each of the wounds in competency 1, tell what signs or symptoms would be cause for concern. How would you deal with each of the concerns?

4. Discuss internal bleeding and how to recognize it (signs and symptoms).

Proficiency Demonstration

1. Develop appropriate subject knowledge through coursework (C), verbal conversation (V), quizzes (Q), worksheets (W), or other approved activities (O).

2. Practice and reinforce the skills in clinical skills and laboratory courses.

3. Refine your skills by observing peer teachers and clinical instructors as they perform the skills (preferably on patients), discussing the competencies with peer teachers and clinical instructors, practicing alone and with others, and then demonstrating proficiency to a peer teacher.

4. Demonstrate your proficiency to an ACI.

APPROVED BY
(date and signature, and mode for didactic)

1a. Abrasion

Didactic _____

Lab _____

Peer _____

ACI _____

1b. Laceration

Didactic _____

Lab _____

Peer _____

ACI _____

1c. Puncture

Didactic _____

Lab _____

Peer _____

ACI _____

1d. Incision

Didactic _____

Lab _____

Peer _____

ACI _____

1e. Avulsion

Didactic _____

Lab _____

Peer _____

ACI _____

2. Wound Care Procedures

2a. Abrasion

Didactic _____

Lab _____

Peer _____

ACI _____

2b. Laceration

Didactic _____

Lab _____

Peer _____

ACI _____

2c. Puncture

Didactic _____

Lab _____

Peer _____

ACI _____

2d. Incision

Didactic _____

Lab _____

Peer _____

ACI _____

2e. Avulsion

Didactic _____

Lab _____

Peer _____

ACI _____

3. Wound Care Anomalies

3a. Abrasion

Didactic _____

Lab _____

Peer _____

ACI _____

3b. Laceration

Didactic _____

Lab _____

Peer _____

ACI _____

3c. Puncture

Didactic _____

Lab _____

Peer _____

ACI _____

3d. Incision

Didactic _____

Lab _____

Peer _____

ACI _____

3e. Avulsion

Didactic _____

Lab _____

Peer _____

ACI _____

4. Internal bleeding

Didactic _____

Lab _____

Peer _____

ACI _____

COMMENTS

_____

_____

_____

_____

_____

_____

_____

_____

_____

_____

Universal Precautions Against Bloodborne Pathogens, Hepatitis, and Tuberculosis

Objective

Understand and be able to apply federal Occupational Health and Safety Administration (OSHA) infection control standards (laws).

NATA Athletic Training Educational Competencies embedded in this module: AD-C7, AC-C13, AC-C15, AC-C28, RM-C2, RM-C6, PA-C5

Competencies

1. Define and discuss OSHA, OSHA standards, and the consequences of ignoring OSHA standards.

2. Define the following:
   a. Bloodborne pathogens
   b. Contaminated laundry
   c. Contaminated sharps
   d. Exposure incidents
   e. Exposure control plan
   f. Hand-washing facilities
   g. Occupational exposure
   h. Other potentially infectious materials
   i. Personal protective equipment
   j. Source individual
   k. Universal precautions
   l. Hepatitis A
   m. Hepatitis B
   n. Hepatitis C
   o. Tuberculosis

3. Locate where the sharps containers, rubber gloves, and isopropyl alcohol or other acceptable disinfectants are kept in each athletic training clinic you will work in during your student career. Discuss the benefits and limitations of these methods of protection.

4. Demonstrate how you would mix an effective solution to disinfect a wrestling mat or examination table of potential human immunodeficiency virus (HIV) contamination after an athlete has bled on it. What would you do with the materials (towels, sponges, and the like) you used to clean the mat?

5. Explain the methods of transmission of HIV and hepatitis B that place allied health care workers at risk. Describe the transmission methods of hepatitis A and hepatitis C and the types of precautions you would take in your role as an AT to protect yourself from transmission.

6. Using a student volunteer and the appropriate supplies and equipment, simulate how you would debride an open (bleeding) wound in an athlete given what you now know about the OSHA guidelines and HIV and hepatitis transmission.

7. Define *tuberculosis* and describe how the disease is spread. Describe the four types of control measures to be taken by health care workers who are at risk for occupational exposure to the disease.

Proficiency Demonstration

1. Develop appropriate subject knowledge through coursework (C), verbal conversation (V), quizzes (Q), worksheets (W), or other approved activities (O).

2. Practice and reinforce the skills in clinical skills and laboratory courses.

3. Refine your skills by observing peer teachers and clinical instructors as they perform the skills (preferably on patients), discussing the competencies with peer teachers and clinical instructors, practicing alone and with others, and then demonstrating proficiency to a peer teacher.

4. Demonstrate your proficiency to an ACI.

APPROVED BY
(date and signature, and mode for didactic)

1. OSHA
   Didactic _____
   Lab _____
   Peer _____
   ACI _____

2. Term definitions
   Didactic _____
   Lab _____
   Peer _____
   ACI _____

3. Equipment location
   Didactic _____
   Lab _____
   Peer _____
   ACI _____

4. Disinfectant solution

Didactic _____

Lab _____

Peer _____

ACI _____

5. Disease transmission

Didactic _____

Lab _____

Peer _____

ACI _____

6. Wound debridement

Didactic _____

Lab _____

Peer _____

ACI _____

7. Tuberculosis and control measures

Didactic _____

Lab _____

Peer _____

ACI _____

COMMENTS

_____

_____

_____

_____

_____

Environmental Injury and Illness

Objective

Develop and demonstrate the skills necessary to recognize and manage selected environment-related injuries and illnesses.

NATA Athletic Training Educational Competencies embedded in this module: RM-C8, RM-C9, RM-C10, RM-C20, RM-P6, RM-CP3, DI-C14, MC-C22, AC-C29, AC-P3, AC-P4, NU-C13

Competencies

1. Discuss the conditions and situations related to the following environmental factors that are potentially hazardous to athletes. Discuss recommendations and position statements for athletic activity to lessen the potential for injury.

 a. Heat
 b. Humidity
 c. Cold
 d. Wind
 e. Lightning strike
 f. Poor air quality

2. Demonstrate and explain the proper use of the following items and how to interpret data from them:

 a. Sling psychrometer
 b. Wet-bulb globe index

3. Explain the signs, symptoms, and management of the following:

 a. Heat cramps
 b. Heat exhaustion
 c. Heat syncope
 d. Heat stroke
 e. Hypothermia

4. Explain physical and environmental factors that are potential hazards for athletes participating in the following activity settings. Tell how and how often you should check each.

 a. Basketball court
 b. American football field
 c. Soccer field
 d. Softball field
 e. Volleyball court

5. Explain how to use and interpret weight charts. For which sports are weight charts most important?

Proficiency Demonstration

1. Develop appropriate subject knowledge through coursework (C), verbal conversation (V), quizzes (Q), worksheets (W), or other approved activities (O).

2. Practice and reinforce the skills in clinical skills and laboratory courses.

3. Refine your skills by observing peer teachers and clinical instructors as they perform the skills (preferably on patients), discussing the competencies with peer teachers and clinical instructors, practicing alone and with others, and then demonstrating proficiency to a peer teacher.

4. Demonstrate your proficiency to an ACI.

APPROVED BY
(date and signature, and mode for didactic)

1. Environmental hazards
 Didactic _____
 Lab _____
 Peer _____
 ACI _____

2. Devices
 Didactic _____
 Lab _____
 Peer _____
 ACI _____

3. Heat-related conditions
 Peer _____
 ACI _____

4. Sport-specific hazards
 Didactic _____
 Lab _____
 Peer _____
 ACI _____

5. Weight charts
 Didactic _____
 Lab _____
 Peer _____
 ACI _____

COMMENTS

_____

Anaphylaxis and Asthma Attacks

Objective

Demonstrate the skills necessary to use epinephrine to treat anaphylaxis and bronchodilators to prevent asthma attacks.

NATA Athletic Training Educational Competencies embedded in this module: MC-C2, MC-C7, MC-C8, MC-C9, AC-C1, AC-C27, AC-P3, AC-P4

Competencies

1. Explain the legal implication of an AT using epinephrine.

2. Demonstrate the ability to use an epinephrine injection in an emergency to treat anaphylaxis:

   a. Identify indications for an epinephrine injection.

   b. Demonstrate verbal and nonverbal instructions necessary to properly use an epinephrine injection.

   c. Identify signs and symptoms associated with an allergic reaction to, or overdose of, epinephrine.

   d. Identify countermeasures you would take if you suspected an allergic reaction to, or overdose of, epinephrine.

   e. Demonstrate proper storage of injectable epinephrine.

   f. Demonstrate proper disposal of a used injection system.

3. Demonstrate the ability to use an emergency bronchodilator inhaler to prevent asthma attacks:

   a. Identify indications for use of a bronchodilator.

   b. Demonstrate verbal and nonverbal instructions to properly use a bronchodilator inhaler.

   c. Identify signs and symptoms associated with an allergic reaction to, or overdose of, a bronchodilator.

   d. Identify countermeasures you would take if you suspected an allergic reaction to, or overdose of, a bronchodilator.

   e. Demonstrate proper storage of a bronchodilator.

Proficiency Demonstration

1. Develop appropriate subject knowledge through coursework (C), verbal conversation (V), quizzes (Q), worksheets (W), or other approved activities (O).

2. Practice and reinforce the skills in clinical skills and laboratory courses.

3. Refine your skills by observing peer teachers and clinical instructors as they perform the skills (preferably on patients), discussing the competencies with peer teachers and clinical instructors, practicing alone and with others, and then demonstrating proficiency to a peer teacher.

4. Demonstrate your proficiency to an ACI.

APPROVED BY
(date and signature, and mode for didactic)

1. Legal implications

   Didactic _____

   Lab _____

   Peer _____

   ACI _____

2. Epinephrine

   Didactic _____

   Lab _____

   Peer _____

   ACI _____

3. Bronchodilator

   Didactic _____

   Lab _____

   Peer _____

   ACI _____

COMMENTS

_____

_____

_____

_____

_____

Poison Control Center

Objective

Demonstrate the skills necessary to report a drug overdose or poisoning to the nearest poison control center.

NATA Athletic Training Educational Competencies embedded in this module: AC-C27, AC-P4, PH-C9, PH-P3, MC-C17

Competencies

1. Locate the phone number and address of the nearest poison control center.

2. Simulate reporting a drug overdose or poisoning situation, including the following:

   a. Name and location of the person making the call
   b. Name and age of the person who has taken the medication
   c. Name and dosage of the drug taken
   d. Time the drug was taken
   e. Signs and symptoms associated with the overdose or poisoning
   f. Vital signs of the person who has taken the medication

Proficiency Demonstration

1. Develop appropriate subject knowledge through coursework (C), verbal conversation (V), quizzes (Q), worksheets (W), or other approved activities (O).

2. Practice and reinforce the skills in clinical skills and laboratory courses.

3. Refine your skills by observing peer teachers and clinical instructors as they perform the skills (preferably on patients), discussing the competencies with peer teachers and clinical instructors, practicing alone and with others, and then demonstrating proficiency to a peer teacher.

4. Demonstrate your proficiency to an ACI.

APPROVED BY

(date and signature, and mode for didactic)

1. Poison control center phone number

   Peer _____

   ACI _____

2. Simulation—reporting a drug overdose or poisoning situation

   Didactic _____

   Lab _____

   Peer _____

   ACI _____

COMMENTS

_____

_____

_____

_____

_____

Level 1.5

O/P Examination 1

Objectives

Demonstrate your mastery of level 1 skills.

Competencies

Complete the comprehensive O/P examination with a score of at least 85%.

Proficiency Demonstration

O/P examination

Date taken _____

Score _____

Approved by _____

Reexamination (if necessary)

Date _____

Score _____

Approved by _____

Individual Athletic Training Skills Development

Students should now understand the basic operations of an athletic training clinic and be prepared to handle most emergencies that typically occur in organized athletics. Now it is time to develop and demonstrate proficiency in a wider range of psychomotor skills necessary for preventing, assessing, caring for, and rehabilitating athletic and sport injuries. The book knowledge must now be applied to actual patient care. This is where the rubber meets the road.

Much of the knowledge and many of the skills presented in courses and labs are basic and stand alone. However, these psychomotor skills are building blocks for the clinical education process where students combine many of these skills in providing multifactorial care for injured patients. It is important to focus on the bigger picture when teaching, studying, and applying the individual modules. Each skill and knowledge module is a component of larger-picture proficiency. The individual skills presented can be combined to create an improved effect, or they may serve as a precursor for additional skills. For example, complete rehabilitation from an injury occurs through correct assessment and diagnosis of an injury, which influences appropriate application of emergency and acute care skills, followed or enhanced by correct therapeutic modality application and therapeutic exercises. Many skills within these areas can be used for various purposes, and understanding the importance of and place for each skill within the larger picture of providing appropriate medical coverage is more important than learning the skill itself. It is of little benefit to a patient if a practitioner knows how to perform a skill but does not know when or where to execute it.

It is also time for more experiential learning as student members of an athletic training staff for sport teams. When appropriate, students should be exposed to the intricacies, nuances, culture, and socialization of multiple sport and employment settings. The clinical experience modules in this section provide an outline for self-directed learning during these experiences.

Note: This text outlines several standard clinical experiences. Individual athletic training programs may have additional customized clinical experience modules based on specific learning opportunities present at their institution or in their community. The modules presented may serve as a guide for creation of individualized clinical experience modules.

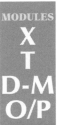

MODULES
X
T
D-M
O/P

There are 92 level 2 modules that are organized into 13 groups, although your program may organize them differently.

- 9 X modules—Directed Clinical Experience (Athletic Training Staff) 53
- 1 T module—Peer Teaching and Supervision 69
- 2 D modules—Surgical Procedures 72
- 4 E modules—The Body. 75
- 9 F modules—Taping, Wrapping, Bracing, and Padding 81
- 6 G modules—Risk Management. 100
- 6 H modules— Basic Nutrition, Pharmacology, and Wellness. 109
- 8 I modules—General Assessment and Evaluation 118
- 12 J modules—Specific Injury Assessment and Diagnosis 131
- 6 K modules—General Medical Conditions, Disorders, and Diseases 194
- 13 L modules—Therapeutic Modalities 209
- 15 M modules—Therapeutic Exercise 229
- 1 O/P module—O/P Examination 2 257

Level 2.1

Directed Clinical Experience (Athletic Training Staff)

Level 1 was designed to introduce students to the practice of athletic training, athletic training clinic operations, and actual patient care. Level 2 clinical experiences allow students to transition from observers to active participants in the health care delivery system. While completing these modules, students will explore, envision, engage, and experience with their clinical instructor the nuances of health care that occur in various venues and sports.

Students begin to participate in independent practice of allowed skills and activities and participate with clinical instructors on more advanced, integrative clinical procedures. In addition to the specific medical knowledge and skills, students should focus on professional behavior, communication, and ethics during their daily interaction with patients, colleagues, coaches, and parents. In addition, emphasis should be placed on understanding the organization of athletic training services, equipment needs, skill development, and the rules and regulations specific to each sport. Every effort should be made to critically examine the similarities and differences between the various venues and sports as athletic training students work on developing and integrating the skills needed to provide appropriate medical care and coverage in varied settings and situations.

Foundational Behaviors of Professional Practice 2

Objective

Discuss how ATs should conduct themselves when acting in a professional capacity, including behavior toward others, such as patients, professional colleagues, coaches and athletic department staff, and the general public.

NATA Athletic Training Educational Competencies embedded in this module: None specifically; these behaviors are to be infused throughout every aspect of the educational program.

Competencies

Define and discuss the following as they relate to how you should conduct yourself as you practice athletic training. Be sure to explain how your thinking and patient interactions have changed during your level 1 clinical experiences.

a. Primacy of the patient

b. Team approach to practice

c. Legal practice

d. Ethical practice

e. Advancing knowledge

f. Cultural competence

g. Professionalism

Proficiency Demonstration

1. Develop appropriate subject knowledge through coursework (C), verbal conversation (V), quizzes (Q), worksheets (W), or other approved activities (O).

2. Demonstrate your proficiency to a peer and to an ACI during clinical experience.

APPROVED BY
(date and signature, and mode for didactic)

1a. Patient primacy

Didactic _____

Lab _____

Peer _____

ACI _____

1b. Team approach

Didactic _____

Lab _____

Peer _____

ACI _____

1c. Legal practice

Didactic _____

Lab _____

Peer _____

ACI _____

1d. Ethical practice

Didactic _____

Lab _____

Peer _____

ACI _____

1e. Knowledge advancement

Didactic _____

Lab _____

Peer _____

ACI _____

1f. Cultural competence

Didactic _____

Lab _____

Peer _____

ACI _____

1g. Professionalism

Didactic _____

Lab _____

Peer _____

ACI _____

COMMENTS

_____

_____

_____

_____

_____

Football Team Experience

NATA Athletic Training Educational Competencies embedded in this module: RM-C1, RM-C9, RM-C16, RM-C17, RM-P4, RM-P5, RM-CP2

Competencies

1. Spend a minimum of 4 weeks as a member of the athletic training staff assigned to an American football team.

2. Outline on paper and discuss with your supervisor the following:

  a. The organization of athletic training services for the football team, including the organization of the athletic training clinic and field (i.e., type of equipment and staff members' functions) for practices and games

  b. Proper fitting of all equipment required by the National Collegiate Athletic Association (NCAA) and the High School Athletic Association (HSAA) and optional equipment for football, including a demonstration of fitting

  c. The skills and activities specific to football that lead to injury

  d. The most common football injuries

  e. Ways to prevent the most common football injuries

  f. NCAA and HSAA rules about taping and bandaging for games

  g. NCAA and HSAA rules about injury care during games

  h. The elements of successful preseason, in-season, and postseason conditioning programs for football, including activities that develop flexibility, strength, muscular endurance, speed, coordination, agility, power, and cardiorespiratory endurance

  i. The three to five athletes on the team who you feel perform their conditioning exercises most correctly, the three to five who perform them least correctly, and why you chose each

Proficiency Demonstration

1. Develop appropriate subject knowledge through coursework (C), verbal conversation (V), quizzes (Q), worksheets (W), or other approved activities (O).

2. Practice and reinforce the skills in clinical skills and laboratory courses.

3. Refine your skills by observing peer teachers and clinical instructors as they perform the skills (preferably on patients), discussing the competencies with peer teachers and clinical instructors, practicing alone and with others, and then demonstrating proficiency to a peer teacher.

4. Demonstrate your proficiency to an ACI.

APPROVED BY
(date and signature, and mode for didactic)

  1. Member of athletic training staff—football

    Peer _____

    ACI _____

  2a. Organization

    Didactic _____

    Lab _____

    Peer _____

    ACI _____

  2b. Equipment

    Didactic _____

    Lab _____

    Peer _____

    ACI _____

  2c. Sport skills

    Didactic _____

    Lab _____

    Peer _____

    ACI _____

  2d. Common injuries

    Didactic _____

    Lab _____

    Peer _____

    ACI _____

  2e. Preventing common injuries

    Didactic _____

    Lab _____

    Peer _____

    ACI _____

2f. Rules about taping

Didactic _____

Lab _____

Peer _____

ACI _____

2g. Rules about injury care

Didactic _____

Lab _____

Peer _____

ACI _____

2h. Conditioning

Didactic _____

Lab _____

Peer _____

ACI _____

2i. Athletes and conditioning exercises

Didactic _____

Lab _____

Peer _____

ACI _____

COMMENTS

_____

_____

_____

_____

_____

Basketball Team Experience

NATA Athletic Training Educational Competencies embedded in this module: RM-C1, RM-C9, RM-C16, RM-C17, RM-P4, RM-P5, RM-CP2

Competencies

1. Spend a minimum of 4 weeks as a member of the athletic training staff assigned to either a men's or women's basketball team.

2. Outline on paper and discuss with your ACI the following:

  a. The organization of athletic training services for the basketball team, including the organization of the athletic training clinic and court (i.e., type of equipment and staff members' functions) for practices and games

  b. Proper fitting of all equipment required by the NCAA and HSAA and optional equipment for basketball, including a demonstration of the fitting

  c. The skills and activities specific to basketball that lead to injury

  d. The most common basketball injuries

  e. Ways to prevent the most common basketball injuries

  f. NCAA and HSAA rules about taping and bandaging for games

  g. NCAA and HSAA rules about injury care during games

  h. The elements of successful preseason, in-season, and postseason conditioning programs for basketball, including activities that develop flexibility, strength, muscular endurance, speed, coordination, agility, power, and cardiorespiratory endurance

  i. The three to five athletes on the team who you feel perform their conditioning exercises most correctly, the three to five who perform them least correctly, and why you chose each

Proficiency Demonstration

1. Develop appropriate subject knowledge through coursework (C), verbal conversation (V), quizzes (Q), worksheets (W), or other approved activities (O).

2. Practice and reinforce the skills in clinical skills and laboratory courses.

3. Refine your skills by observing peer teachers and clinical instructors as they perform the skills (preferably on patients), discussing the competencies with peer teachers and clinical instructors, practicing alone and with others, and then demonstrating proficiency to a peer teacher.

4. Demonstrate your proficiency to an ACI.

APPROVED BY
(date and signature, and mode for didactic)

1. Member of athletic training staff—basketball
ACI _____

2a. Organization
Peer _____
ACI _____

2b. Equipment
Peer _____
ACI _____

2c. Sport skills
Didactic _____
Lab _____
Peer _____
ACI _____

2d. Common injuries
Didactic _____
Lab _____
Peer _____
ACI _____

2e. Preventing common injuries
Didactic _____
Lab _____
Peer _____
ACI _____

2f. Rules about taping
Didactic _____
Lab _____
Peer _____
ACI _____

2g. Rules about injury care

Didactic _____

Lab _____

Peer _____

ACI _____

2h. Conditioning

Didactic _____

Lab _____

Peer _____

ACI _____

2i. Athletes and conditioning exercises

Didactic _____

Lab _____

Peer _____

ACI _____

COMMENTS

_____

_____

_____

_____

_____

_____

_____

_____

NATA Athletic Training Educational Competencies embedded in this module: RM-C1, RM-C9, RM-C16, RM-C17, RM-P4, RM-P5, RM-CP2

Competencies

1. Spend a minimum of 4 weeks as a member of the athletic training staff assigned to a men's team sport (other than football or basketball).

2. Outline on paper and discuss with your ACI the following:

    a. The organization of athletic training services for the team, including the organization of the athletic training clinic and the court or field (i.e., type of equipment and staff members' functions) for practices and games

    b. Proper fitting of all equipment required by the NCAA and HSAA and optional equipment for the team, including a demonstration of the fitting

    c. The skills and activities specific to the sport that lead to injury

    d. The most common injuries in the sport

    e. Ways to prevent the most common injuries in the sport

    f. NCAA and HSAA rules about taping and bandaging for sport contests

    g. NCAA and HSAA rules about injury care during sport contests

    h. Differences from an athletic training point of view between this sport and other sports you have worked with

    i. The elements of successful preseason, in-season, and postseason conditioning programs for this sport, including activities that develop flexibility, strength, muscular endurance, speed, coordination, agility, power, and cardiorespiratory endurance

    j. The three to five athletes on the team who you feel perform their conditioning exercises most correctly, the three to five who perform them least correctly, and why you chose each

Proficiency Demonstration

1. Develop appropriate subject knowledge through coursework (C), verbal conversation (V), quizzes (Q), worksheets (W), or other approved activities (O).

2. Practice and reinforce the skills in clinical skills and laboratory courses.

3. Refine your skills by observing peer teachers and clinical instructors as they perform the skills (preferably on patients), discussing the competencies with peer teachers and clinical instructors, practicing alone and with others, and then demonstrating proficiency to a peer teacher.

4. Demonstrate your proficiency to an ACI.

APPROVED BY
(date and signature, and mode for didactic)

    1. Member of athletic training staff—men's team sport

    ACI _____

  2a. Organization

    Peer _____

    ACI _____

  2b. Equipment

    Peer _____

    ACI _____

  2c. Sport skills

    Didactic _____

    Lab _____

    Peer _____

    ACI_____

  2d. Common injuries

    Didactic _____

    Lab _____

    Peer _____

    ACI _____

  2e. Preventing common injuries

    Didactic _____

    Lab _____

    Peer _____

    ACI _____

  2f. Rules about taping

    Didactic _____

    Lab _____

    Peer _____

    ACI _____

2g. Rules about injury care

Didactic _____

Lab _____

Peer _____

ACI _____

2h. Differences between this sport and others

Didactic _____

Lab _____

Peer _____

ACI _____

2i. Conditioning

Didactic _____

Lab _____

Peer _____

ACI _____

2j. Athletes and conditioning exercises

Didactic _____

Lab _____

Peer _____

ACI _____

COMMENTS

_____

_____

_____

_____

_____

Women's Team Sport Experience

NATA Athletic Training Educational Competencies embedded in this module: RM-C1, RM-C9, RM-C16, RM-C17, RM-P4, RM-P5, RM-CP2

Competencies

1. Spend a minimum of 4 weeks as a member of the athletic training staff assigned to a women's team sport (other than basketball).

2. Outline on paper and discuss with your ACI the following:

a. The organization of athletic training services for the team, including the organization of the athletic training clinic and the court or field (i.e., type of equipment and staff members' functions) for practices and games

b. Proper fitting of all equipment required by the NCAA and HSAA and optional equipment for the team, including a demonstration of the fitting

c. The skills and activities specific to the sport that lead to injury

d. The most common injuries in the sport

e. Ways to prevent the most common injuries in the sport

f. NCAA and HSAA rules about taping and bandaging for sport contests

g. NCAA and HSAA rules about injury care during sport contests

h. Differences from an athletic training point of view between this sport and other sports you have worked with

i. The elements of successful preseason, in-season, and postseason conditioning programs for this sport, including activities that develop flexibility, strength, muscular endurance, speed, coordination, agility, power, and cardiorespiratory endurance

j. The three to five athletes on the team who you feel perform their conditioning exercises most correctly, the three to five who perform them least correctly, and why you chose each

Proficiency Demonstration

1. Develop appropriate subject knowledge through coursework (C), verbal conversation (V), quizzes (Q), worksheets (W), or other approved activities (O).

2. Practice and reinforce the skills in clinical skills and laboratory courses.

3. Refine your skills by observing peer teachers and clinical instructors as they perform the skills (preferably on patients), discussing the competencies with peer teachers and clinical instructors, practicing alone and with others, and then demonstrating proficiency to a peer teacher.

4. Demonstrate your proficiency to an ACI.

APPROVED BY
(date and signature, and mode for didactic)

1. Member of athletic training staff—women's team sport

ACI _____

2a. Organization

Peer _____

ACI _____

2b. Equipment

Peer _____

ACI _____

2c. Sport skills

Didactic _____

Lab _____

Peer _____

ACI _____

2d. Common injuries

Didactic _____

Lab _____

Peer _____

ACI _____

2e. Preventing common injuries

Didactic _____

Lab _____

Peer _____

ACI _____

2f. Rules about taping

Didactic _____

Lab _____

Peer _____

ACI _____

2g. Rules about injury care

Didactic _____

Lab _____

Peer _____

ACI _____

2h. Differences between this sport and others

Didactic _____

Lab _____

Peer _____

ACI _____

2i. Conditioning

Didactic _____

Lab _____

Peer _____

ACI _____

2j. Athletes and conditioning exercises

Didactic _____

Lab _____

Peer _____

ACI _____

COMMENTS

_____

_____

_____

_____

_____

Men's Individual Sport Experience

NATA Athletic Training Educational Competencies embedded in this module: RM-C1, RM-C9, RM-C16, RM-C17, RM-P4, RM-P5, RM-CP2

Competencies

1. Spend a minimum of 4 weeks as a member of the athletic training staff for a men's team that involves individual sport competition (e.g., gymnastics, track and field).

2. Outline on paper and discuss with your ACI the following:

   a. The organization of athletic training services for the team, including the organization of the athletic training clinic and the court or field (i.e., type of equipment and staff members' functions) for practices and games
   b. Proper fitting of all equipment required by the NCAA and HSAA and optional equipment for the team, including a demonstration of the fitting
   c. The skills and activities specific to the sport that lead to injury
   d. The most common injuries in the sport
   e. Ways to prevent the most common injuries in the sport
   f. NCAA and HSAA rules about taping and bandaging for sport contests
   g. NCAA and HSAA rules about injury care during sport contests
   h. Differences from an athletic training point of view between this sport and other sports you have worked with
   i. The elements of successful preseason, in-season, and postseason conditioning programs for this sport, including activities that develop flexibility, strength, muscular endurance, speed, coordination, agility, power, and cardiorespiratory endurance
   j. The three to five athletes on the team who you feel perform their conditioning exercises most correctly, the three to five who perform them least correctly, and why you chose each

Proficiency Demonstration

1. Develop appropriate subject knowledge through coursework (C), verbal conversation (V), quizzes (Q), worksheets (W), or other approved activities (O).

2. Practice and reinforce the skills in clinical skills and laboratory courses.

3. Refine your skills by observing peer teachers and clinical instructors as they perform the skills (preferably on patients), discussing the competencies with peer teachers and clinical instructors, practicing alone and with others, and then demonstrating proficiency to a peer teacher.

4. Demonstrate your proficiency to an ACI.

APPROVED BY
(date and signature, and mode for didactic)

1. Member of athletic training staff—men's individual sport
   ACI _____

2a. Organization
   Peer _____
   ACI _____

2b. Equipment
   Peer _____
   ACI _____

2c. Sport skills
   Didactic _____
   Lab _____
   Peer _____
   ACI _____

2d. Common injuries
   Didactic _____
   Lab _____
   Peer _____
   ACI _____

2e. Preventing common injuries
   Didactic _____
   Lab _____
   Peer _____
   ACI _____

2f. Rules about taping

Didactic _____

Lab _____

Peer _____

ACI _____

2g. Rules about injury care

Didactic _____

Lab _____

Peer _____

ACI _____

2h. Differences between this sport and others

Didactic _____

Lab _____

Peer _____

ACI _____

2i. Conditioning

Didactic _____

Lab _____

Peer _____

ACI _____

2j. Athletes and conditioning exercises

Didactic _____

Lab _____

Peer _____

ACI _____

COMMENTS

_____

_____

_____

_____

_____

_____

_____

_____

Women's Individual Sport Experience

NATA Athletic Training Educational Competencies embedded in this module: RM-C1, RM-C9, RM-C16, RM-C17, RM-P4, RM-P5, RM-CP2

Competencies

1. Spend a minimum of 4 weeks as a member of the athletic training staff for a women's team that involves individual sport competition (e.g., gymnastics, track and field).

2. Outline on paper and discuss with your ACI the following:

   a. The organization of athletic training services for the team, including the organization of the athletic training clinic and the court or field (i.e., type of equipment and staff members' functions) for practices and games.
   b. Proper fitting of all equipment required by the NCAA and HSAA and optional equipment for the team, including a demonstration of the fitting
   c. The skills and activities specific to the sport that lead to injury
   d. The most common injuries in the sport
   e. Ways to prevent the most common injuries in the sport
   f. NCAA and HSAA rules about taping and bandaging for sport contests
   g. NCAA and HSAA rules about injury care during sport contests
   h. Differences from an athletic training point of view between this sport and other sports you have worked with
   i. The elements of successful preseason, in-season, and postseason conditioning programs for this sport, including activities that develop flexibility, strength, muscular endurance, speed, coordination, agility, power, and cardiorespiratory endurance
   j. The three to five athletes on the team who you feel perform their conditioning exercises most correctly, the three to five who perform them least correctly, and why you chose each

Proficiency Demonstration

1. Develop appropriate subject knowledge through coursework (C), verbal conversation (V), quizzes (Q), worksheets (W), or other approved activities (O).

2. Practice and reinforce the skills in clinical skills and laboratory courses.

3. Refine your skills by observing peer teachers and clinical instructors as they perform the skills (preferably on patients), discussing the competencies with peer teachers and clinical instructors, practicing alone and with others, and then demonstrating proficiency to a peer teacher.

4. Demonstrate your proficiency to an ACI.

APPROVED BY
(date and signature, and mode for didactic)

1. Member of athletic training staff—women's individual sport
   ACI _____

2a. Organization
   Peer _____
   ACI _____

2b. Equipment
   Peer _____
   ACI _____

2c. Sport skills
   Didactic _____
   Lab _____
   Peer _____
   ACI _____

2d. Common injuries
   Didactic _____
   Lab _____
   Peer _____
   ACI _____

2e. Preventing common injuries
   Didactic _____
   Lab _____
   Peer _____
   ACI _____

2f. Rules about taping
   Didactic _____
   Lab _____
   Peer _____
   ACI _____

2g. Rules about injury care

Didactic _____

Lab _____

Peer _____

ACI _____

2h. Differences between this sport and others

Didactic _____

Lab _____

Peer _____

ACI _____

2i. Conditioning

Didactic _____

Lab _____

Peer _____

ACI _____

2j. Athletes and conditioning exercises

Didactic _____

Lab _____

Peer _____

ACI _____

COMMENTS

_____

_____

_____

_____

_____

High School Experience

NATA Athletic Training Educational Competencies embedded in this module: RM-C1, RM-C9, RM-C16, RM-C17, RM-P4, RM-P5, RM-CP2

Competencies

1. Spend a minimum of 4 weeks as a member of the athletic training staff for a high school.

2. Outline on paper and discuss with your ACI the following:

    a. The organization of athletic training services for the school, including the organization of the athletic training clinic and the court or field (i.e., type of equipment and staff members' functions) for practices and games

    b. Role of parents and personal physicians in care of the juvenile athlete's injuries and illnesses

    c. Differences between juveniles and adults in how they deal with pain

    d. Injuries and illnesses that are more prevalent in juveniles than in college athletes

    e. Injuries and illnesses that are less prevalent in juveniles than in college athletes

    f. Time spent treating injuries

    g. Differences from an athletic training point of view between high school and college athletics

Proficiency Demonstration

1. Develop appropriate subject knowledge through coursework (C), verbal conversation (V), quizzes (Q), worksheets (W), or other approved activities (O).

2. Practice and reinforce the skills in clinical skills and laboratory courses.

3. Refine your skills by observing peer teachers and clinical instructors as they perform the skills (preferably on patients), discussing the competencies with peer teachers and clinical instructors, practicing alone and with others, and then demonstrating proficiency to a peer teacher.

4. Demonstrate your proficiency to an ACI.

APPROVED BY
(date and signature, and mode for didactic)

1. Member of athletic training staff—high school

    ACI _____

2a. Organization

    Peer _____

    ACI _____

2b. Role of parents and personal physicians

    Peer _____

    ACI _____

2c. Sport skills

    Didactic _____

    Lab _____

    Peer _____

    ACI _____

2d. Injuries that are more prevalent among juveniles

    Didactic _____

    Lab _____

    Peer _____

    ACI _____

2e. Injuries that are less prevalent among juveniles

    Didactic _____

    Lab _____

    Peer _____

    ACI _____

2f. Time for treating injuries

    Didactic _____

    Lab _____

    Peer _____

    ACI _____

2g. Differences between high school and college athletics

    Didactic _____

    Lab _____

    Peer _____

    ACI _____

COMMENTS

_____

_____

Sports Medicine Clinic or Industrial Experience

NATA Athletic Training Educational Competencies embedded in this module: RM-C1

Competencies

1. Spend a minimum of 4 weeks as a member of the athletic training staff in a sports medicine or industrial health clinic.

2. Outline on paper and discuss with your ACI the following:

    a. The organization of athletic training services of the clinic, including the organization in the clinic and any outreach services provided (i.e., type of equipment and staff members' functions)

    b. The most common injuries seen in the clinic

    c. Things patients could do to prevent the most common injuries

    d. Differences between working in a sports medicine clinic and a college or high school athletic training department

Proficiency Demonstration

1. Develop appropriate subject knowledge through coursework (C), verbal conversation (V), quizzes (Q), worksheets (W), or other approved activities (O).

2. Practice and reinforce the skills in clinical skills and laboratory courses.

3. Refine your skills by observing peer teachers and clinical instructors as they perform the skills (preferably on patients), discussing the competencies with peer teachers and clinical instructors, practicing alone and with others, and then demonstrating proficiency to a peer teacher.

4. Demonstrate your proficiency to an ACI.

APPROVED BY
(date and signature, and mode for didactic)

1. Member of athletic training staff—sports medicine or industrial health clinic

    ACI _____

2a. Organization

    Peer _____

    ACI _____

2b. Common conditions

    Peer _____

    ACI _____

2c. Preventing common conditions

    Peer _____

    ACI _____

2d. Difference between settings

    Didactic _____

    Lab _____

    Peer _____

    ACI _____

COMMENTS

_____

_____

_____

_____

_____

_____

Level 2.2

Peer Teaching and Supervision

Peer teaching can be likened to good parenting. Parents have been known to provide much instruction and sacrifice for their children, with the only expectation for payment being the hope that the same actions will be provided to future generations. This is essentially what is expected from participating in the peer teaching modules. Previously taught by peers, it is now time for students to instruct those who follow.

The biblical adage "it is better to give than to receive" holds special meaning when it comes to peer teaching. Often the teacher (giver) gains the most benefit from this instructional tutoring, although both parties certainly benefit.

Peer teaching level 1 students is an opportunity for level 2 students to provide instruction on the basic skills presented in the level 1 modules (*Athletic Training Clinic Operations* and *Emergency and Acute Care of Injuries and Illnesses*). Peer teachers benefit those whom they teach, and benefit themselves by reviewing and deepening their own knowledge of the subject.

Teaching can only be done with an appropriate knowledge base from which to draw upon. Preparation prior to a peer teaching session is critical for appropriate delivery and application of the information.

Review the *Peer Teaching for Deeper Learning* in chapter 1 before you begin. Remember, it is OK to not immediately know the answer to a question, but it is *not* acceptable to ignore it. Both the peer student and peer teacher need to be active participants in the process of peer teaching. Learn together and learn from each other.

Teaching Level 1 Athletic Training Students

Objective

Teach and assess mastery of level 1 students, and deepen your own understanding and mastery of those skills.

Competencies

1. Peer teach at least five level 1 students and at least 15 level 1 modules. This includes reviewing material with the students, offering suggestions and corrections as they practice the skills, and assessing their mastery of the skill when appropriate. Students must practice the skills enough to become proficient in them before the assessment. Refer often to references and teaching aids.

2. Discuss your peer teaching experience with a faculty athletic trainer or ACI.

Proficiency Demonstration

1. Record your peer teaching experiences in the spaces provided.

Name of student	Module	Review date	Assessment date
1.			
2.			
3.			
4.			
5.			
6.			
7.			
8.			
9.			
10.			
11.			
12.			
13.			
14.			
15.			
16.			
17.			
18.			
19.			
20.			
21.			
22.			
23.			
24.			

Name of student	Module	Review date	Assessment date
25. _____	_____	_____	_____
26. _____	_____	_____	_____
27. _____	_____	_____	_____
28. _____	_____	_____	_____
29. _____	_____	_____	_____
30. _____	_____	_____	_____

2. Task completed and discussed (date)

Peer _____

ACI _____

COMMENTS

_____

_____

_____

Surgical Procedures

Rehabilitating patients following surgery is a major responsibility of athletic trainers. Understanding surgical procedures and techniques enhances the athletic trainer's rehabilitation skills. These two modules expose students to general surgical principles, specific techniques of selected surgical procedures, and the operating room during surgery.

Basic Surgical Procedures

Objective

Develop an understanding of objectives, procedures, and implications for rehabilitation of common corrective orthopedic procedures.

NATA Athletic Training Educational Competencies embedded in this module: AC-C16, AC-C30, AC-C31, EX-C3

Competencies

1. Describe basic preoperative surgical procedures performed in the physician's office or hospital operating room.

2. Describe basic postoperative surgical procedures, including hospital care and discharge recommendations.

3. Describe the purpose, procedures, and rehabilitative challenges of an anterior cruciate ligament (ACL) surgery of your choice.

4. Describe the purpose, procedures, and rehabilitative challenges of a shoulder surgery of your choice.

5. Describe the purpose, procedures, and rehabilitative challenges of an open reduction internal fixation (ORIF) surgery of your choice.

6. Describe the purpose, procedures, and rehabilitative challenges of a chest, spine, or trunk surgery of your choice.

Proficiency Demonstration

1. Develop appropriate subject knowledge through coursework (C), verbal conversation (V), quizzes (Q), worksheets (W), or other approved activities (O).

2. Practice and reinforce the skills in clinical skills and laboratory courses.

3. Refine your skills by observing peer teachers and clinical instructors as they perform the skills (preferably on patients), discussing the competencies with peer teachers and clinical instructors, practicing alone and with others, and then demonstrating proficiency to a peer teacher.

4. Demonstrate your proficiency to an ACI.

APPROVED BY

(date and signature, and mode for didactic)

1. Preoperative procedures

Didactic _____

Lab _____

Peer _____

ACI _____

2. Postoperative procedures

Didactic _____

Lab _____

Peer _____

ACI _____

3. ACL surgery: _____

Didactic _____

Lab _____

Peer _____

ACI _____

4. Shoulder surgery: _____

Didactic _____

Lab _____

Peer _____

ACI _____

5. ORIF surgery: _____

Didactic _____

Lab _____

Peer _____

ACI _____

6. Chest, spine, or trunk surgery: _____

Didactic _____

Lab _____

Peer _____

ACI _____

COMMENTS

_____

_____

_____

_____

Surgical Observation

Objective

Develop an appreciation for what athletes go through during surgery. Note: J modules can be completed simultaneously with this module.

NATA Athletic Training Educational Competencies embedded in this module: none

Competencies

1. Observe two different surgical procedures. With each, discuss with a physician, surgical nurse, or technician the presurgical preparation of the patient and the procedures that will be followed for the 12 to 24 hours after surgery.

2. Within 48 hours of the surgery (the sooner the better), discuss the surgery with a peer and an ACI. Include in this discussion the rehabilitation procedures that this patient probably will follow.

Proficiency Demonstration

1. Surgery 1

Patient _____

Procedure _____

Date _____

Physician _____

2. Surgery 2

Athlete _____

Procedure _____

Date _____

Physician _____

APPROVED BY (DATE AND SIGNATURE)

Peer _____

ACI _____

COMMENTS

_____

_____

_____

_____

_____

_____

Level 2.4

The Body

By definition, an athletic trainer is a health care professional who works with an active population, and it therefore stands to reason that knowledge of the body, human development, physiology, pathology, and hygiene is foundational to the framework of athletic training education. Similar to other health care professions, certain information must be understood before proceeding to more advanced information and skills. We must walk before we run.

The modules that explore body systems and development, exercise for the young and old, physiology of exercise, trauma response, injury and illness pathology, and current concepts in health and wellness have been placed in level 2 as part of basic knowledge and skills. This is because as members of the athletic training profession, we are expected to be confident in our knowledge of the information presented in these modules. The information in the following modules affects acute care, assessment and evaluation, treatment, rehabilitation, performance enhancement, and healthy lifestyle choices. Being able to share, teach, explain, and use this information to guide and inform decisions is critical to providing appropriate medical care. Because this information is foundational, students must be sure they are completely comfortable with the knowledge required of these modules before moving on to more advanced modules. Students should work with their faculty instructors and ACIs to make sure they understand this information at a satisfactory level before proceeding.

Body Systems and Development

Objective

Develop and demonstrate a working knowledge of the body systems and the impact of athletic activity throughout a lifetime.

NATA Athletic Training Educational Competencies embedded in this module: DI-C1, DI-C2

Systems for This Module

Cardiovascular

Respiratory

Immune

Endocrine

Digestive

Urinary and excretory

Nervous

Reproductive

Integumentary

Musculoskeletal

Competencies

1. Demonstrate knowledge of the anatomy, purpose, and function of the body systems listed previously.

2. For each of the listed body systems, summarize the anatomical and physiological development that occurs throughout a person's lifetime.

3. Demonstrate knowledge of the basic principles associated with motor development and other development characteristics.

4. Demonstrate knowledge of the Tanner stages of sexual development.

Proficiency Demonstration

1. Develop appropriate subject knowledge through coursework (C), verbal conversation (V), quizzes (Q), worksheets (W), or other approved activities (O).

2. Practice and reinforce the skills in clinical skills and laboratory courses.

3. Refine your skills by observing peer teachers and clinical instructors as they perform the skills (preferably on patients), discussing the competencies with peer teachers and clinical instructors, practicing alone and with others, and then demonstrating proficiency to a peer teacher.

4. Demonstrate your proficiency to an ACI.

APPROVED BY
(date and signature, and mode for didactic)

1. Body systems anatomy and function

Didactic _____

Lab _____

Peer _____

ACI _____

2. Anatomical development

Didactic _____

Lab _____

Peer _____

ACI _____

3. Motor development

Didactic _____

Lab _____

Peer _____

ACI _____

4. Tanner stages

Didactic _____

Lab _____

Peer _____

ACI _____

COMMENTS

_____

_____

_____

_____

_____

_____

_____

Injury and Illness Pathology

Objective

Develop and demonstrate knowledge regarding the normal pathological processes within the human body and how these processes are affected during injury or illness.

NATA Athletic Training Educational Competencies embedded in this module: PA-C1, PA-C2, PA-C3, PA-C4, PA-C5, PA-C6

Competencies

1. Describe normal cellular structure and function and adaptations due to acute and chronic stress; changes due to injury, illness, and disease; and the symptoms associated with these changes.

2. Describe the physiology of circulation and fluid homeostasis and changes that occur due to acute and chronic stress and following injury, illness, and disease.

3. Describe the etiology, pathogenesis, pathomechanics, signs, symptoms, and epidemiology of the following:

a. Musculoskeletal injury
   1. Fracture
   2. Soft tissue contusion
   3. Soft tissue strain
   4. Soft tissue sprain
b. Illness
   1. Acute upper-respiratory infection
   2. Acute lower-respiratory infection
   3. Chronic upper-respiratory infection
   4. Chronic lower-respiratory infection
   5. Influenza
   6. Mononucleosis
   7. Bacterial and viral infections
c. Disease
   1. Asthma
   2. Diabetes
   3. Sickle cell trait
d. Aging
e. Medications
   1. Blockers
   2. Stimulants
   3. Depressants
f. Nutritional deficiencies
   1. Anemia
   2. Vitamin B$_{12}$
   3. Anorexia nervosa
   4. Bulimia
   5. Restricted eating

Proficiency Demonstration

1. Develop appropriate subject knowledge through coursework (C), verbal conversation (V), quizzes (Q), worksheets (W), or other approved activities (O).

2. Refine your knowledge through discussions with peer teachers and clinical instructors.

3. Demonstrate proficiency to a peer teacher and an ACI.

APPROVED BY
(date and signature, and mode for didactic)

1. Understanding cells

Didactic _____

Peer _____

ACI _____

2. Circulatory and fluid physiology

Didactic _____

Peer _____

ACI _____

3. Physiological and pathological responses

Didactic _____

Peer _____

ACI _____

COMMENTS

_____

_____

_____

_____

Exercise and Disease

Objective

Develop and demonstrate understanding of the physiological responses of the human body experiences during and following exercise in hot or cold environments, as well as with common illnesses, abnormalities, and diseases.

NATA Athletic Training Educational Competencies embedded in this module: DI-C1, DI-C3, MC-C1, MC-C2

Competencies

1. Demonstrate knowledge and understanding of how exercise affects, both acutely and chronically, the normal physiology of the following systems of the human body:

    a. Cardiovascular
    b. Respiratory
    c. Nervous
    d. Musculoskeletal
    e. Thermoregulatory
    f. Digestive
    g. Reproductive

2. Describe the physiological effects of the following common illnesses, abnormalities, and diseases on the body systems listed in competency 1, including the effect these changes have on exercise and performance. Include when you would refer patients of all ages with these conditions to other medial and health care professionals and to whom you would refer them.

    a. Rhinovirus
    b. Influenza
    c. Upper respiratory infection
    d. Lower-respiratory infection
    e. Diabetes
    f. Arthritis
    g. Exercise-induced asthma
    h. Vocal cord dysfunction
    i. Irritable bowel syndrome or Crohn's disease
    j. Blood clotting disorders
    k. Stomach ulcers
    l. Ovarian cysts
    m. Amenorrhea or oligomenorrhea
    n. Single-paired organs

Proficiency Demonstration

1. Develop appropriate subject knowledge through coursework (C), verbal conversation (V), quizzes (Q), worksheets (W), or other approved activities (O).

2. Refine your knowledge through discussions with peer teachers and clinical instructors.

3. Demonstrate proficiency to a peer teacher and an ACI.

APPROVED BY
(date and signature, and mode for didactic)

1a. Cardiovascular

    Didactic _____

    Peer _____

    ACI _____

1b. Respiratory

    Didactic _____

    Peer _____

    ACI _____

1c. Nervous

    Didactic _____

    Peer _____

    ACI _____

1d. Musculoskeletal

    Didactic _____

    Peer _____

    ACI _____

1e. Thermoregulatory

    Didactic _____

    Peer _____

    ACI _____

1f. Digestive

    Didactic _____

    Peer _____

    ACI _____

1g. Reproductive

Didactic _____

Peer _____

ACI _____

2a. Rhinovirus

Didactic _____

Peer _____

ACI _____

2b. Influenza

Didactic _____

Peer _____

ACI _____

2c. Upper respiratory infection

Didactic _____

Peer _____

ACI _____

2d. Lower-respiratory infection

Didactic _____

Peer _____

ACI _____

2e. Diabetes

Didactic _____

Peer _____

ACI _____

2f. Arthritis

Didactic _____

Peer _____

ACI _____

2g. Exercise-induced asthma

Didactic _____

Peer _____

ACI _____

2h. Vocal cord dysfunction

Didactic _____

Peer _____

ACI _____

2i. Irritable bowel syndrome or Crohn's disease

Didactic _____

Peer _____

ACI _____

2j. Blood clotting disorders

Didactic _____

Peer _____

ACI _____

2k. Stomach ulcers

Didactic _____

Peer _____

ACI _____

2l. Ovarian cysts

Didactic _____

Peer _____

ACI _____

2m. Amenorrhea or oligomenorrhea

Didactic _____

Peer _____

ACI _____

2n. Single-paired organs

Didactic _____

Peer _____

ACI _____

COMMENTS

_____

_____

_____

_____

_____

_____

Objective

Develop an understanding of the physiological, pathological, and psychological processes that occur within the body in response to trauma.

NATA Athletic Training Educational Competencies embedded in this module: AC-C18, PA-C4, TM-C1, TM-C4

Competencies

1. Describe the pathophysiology of the inflammatory process as it occurs following invasion of microbiologic agents and acute and chronic injury.

2. Describe the signs and symptoms of acute and chronic inflammation.

3. Describe the pathophysiology of wound healing and tissue repair.

4. Discuss the effects of genetic derangements, nutritional deficiencies, chemicals, drugs, and aging on inflammation and wound repair.

5. Discuss the effects of disuse on the musculoskeletal system and other organ systems.

6. Discuss the use of therapeutic modalities for promoting acute wound repair.

7. Describe the psychophysiology of pain and relevant theories of pain perception.

8. Discuss techniques of measuring pain

9. Discuss techniques of managing acute and chronic (persistent) pain.

Proficiency Demonstration

1. Develop appropriate subject knowledge through coursework (C), verbal conversation (V), quizzes (Q), worksheets (W), or other approved activities (O).

2. Refine your knowledge through discussions with peer teachers and clinical instructors.

3. Demonstrate proficiency to a peer teacher and an ACI.

APPROVED BY
(date and signature, and mode for didactic)

1. Inflammatory process

    Didactic _____

    Lab _____

    Peer _____

    ACI _____

2. Signs and symptoms

    Didactic _____

    Lab _____

    Peer _____

    ACI _____

3. Wound healing

    Didactic _____

    Peer _____

    ACI _____

4. Effects on inflammation and wound repair

    Didactic _____

    Peer _____

    ACI _____

5. Effects of disuse

    Didactic _____

    Peer _____

    ACI _____

6. Therapeutic modalities

    Didactic _____

    Peer _____

    ACI _____

7. Pain and theories

    Didactic _____

    Peer _____

    ACI _____

8. Measuring pain

    Didactic _____

    Peer _____

    ACI _____

9. Managing pain

    Didactic _____

    Peer _____

    ACI _____

COMMENTS

_____

_____

Taping, Wrapping, Bracing, and Padding

It is impossible to determine which of the many skills and responsibilities performed by ATs is most vital to the profession. Tapping, wrapping, and bandaging skills, however, are probably the most often used and definitely the most visible. Right or wrong, others may perceive the competence of ATs based solely on how well they tape, wrap, and bandage. These experiences are often an AT's first intensive and personal contact with an athlete.

It is reasonable to assume that ATs will spend significant time learning, practicing, and performing these important skills during their career. Although many of the techniques are specific to body parts, there are a few methods of tape and wrap application that can be slightly modified to achieve a desired effect.

Tape or wraps are applied at various times during patient care. Medical care goals must be constantly examined to see if tape can facilitate prevention, immediate care, treatment, or rehabilitation of patients. These decisions are often based on several factors or desired outcomes. There will be times when the AT feels that compression, support, protection, or restriction of various body parts may facilitate or perhaps limit the movements and function of the parts. These factors determine the type of tape and method of application to be used. It is critical for ATs to determine their treatment objective for each situation and choose the tape, wrap, and method of application accordingly.

Tape can be used as an emergency care technique, a preventative measure, a treatment modality, or a rehabilitative tool. By thinking about the use of tape during all phases of care for the physically active, the AT is taking advantage of a specific skill that is commonly used in the profession.

The following methods of tape, wrap, and bandage application are foundational for the AT and can be applied to many situations and body parts to achieve the desired outcomes. They can be applied as individual techniques, in combination with each other, or with additional methods that are more specific. Creativity with taping techniques and supplies is a valuable skill for ATs as various injuries and taping objectives are encountered.

■ Spiral—Spiral taping is typically used when the AT feels that compression or general support of joints or soft tissue is the objective. Spiral taping and wrapping can also be used in bandaging and wound care. It consists of overlapping layers of tape or wrapping material; the amount of overlapping depends on the taping objectives. Spiral taping for compression and support can be applied either over a joint or long bones and muscle tissue. In most cases it should be applied in a distal-to-proximal fashion to aid in venous return and function. Spiral taping is commonly used for injuries to the thigh, hamstring, quadriceps, lower leg, and wrist, but the technique can be applied to many situations where the benefits of spiral taping meet the treatment objectives.

■ Check reigns—A check reign is a method of taping in which strips of tape cross over a joint in an effort to limit or modify joint movement and protect soft tissue structures. The check reign typically involves anchor strips placed proximal and distal to the involved joint. These anchor strips serve as attachment points for the check reign and can take on several shapes or styles, including stacks, Y, double Y, fan, or X. The main premise behind the check reign is to limit either normal or excessive movement. Length and type of the check reign, application technique, and joint position are all methods the AT can use to produce the desired effect of modifying movement and protecting soft tissue.

– Stacks—A stack check reign is made when strips of tape are placed directly on top of each other in an attempt to strengthen the check reign. The number of strips and subsequently the strength of the check reign are based on the taping objective. Stack check reigns for the knee should typically be stronger than those used on the wrist, but they can be modified to each situation. Stacks can be made from several materials, including cloth tape, elastic tape, neoprene rolls, elastic bands, and cotton or nylon strapping. Toes, knees, elbows, ankles, and fingers are common sites for this application.

– Fan—The fan check reign is similar to the stack check reign except that it is formed so that one end is wider than the other. Overlapping the tape in this way allows for taping to occur over a joint where either the proximal or distal aspect is larger than the other. The fan technique allows for greater contact area, thus creating greater control of motion and support.

– X check reign—This technique uses a crisscross stack or fan to obtain greater contact and control of the joint and soft tissue. This method is often used on areas such as the wrist where the joint is smaller than the distal and proximal aspects of that joint. Narrowing the check reign in the middle allows for less bulk and increased control.

– Y check reign—This style of check reign consists of a stack check reign that is cut or split at one end to facilitate attachment to the anchor strips. The split end of the Y check reign can be made long enough to be placed in a circular fashion around the anchor strip and body part and taped in place. This helps keep the check reign from moving or loosening during activity or participation. The Y check reign is often applied during taping procedures with the aim of limiting ankle movement.

– Double Y check reign—The double Y is a stack check reign with a split on each end. Its purpose is to improve attachment at both anchor sites.

■ Figure eight—The figure-eight taping technique is a foundational technique that can be applied in numerous situations and joints. The figure-eight technique is used to limit motion or provide support for a joint. It involves continuous circular and angular placement of the tape so that it crosses over itself and the joint while circumnavigating the proximal and distal aspects of the bones of the joint. Tape tension, joint placement while taping, and type of tape are factors that influence the restrictive and supportive nature of this procedure. This technique is applied to the ankles, wrists, fingers, elbows, shoulders, hips, and knees.

Note: The aforementioned taping techniques are foundational and can be used in isolation or in conjunction with each other in a taping procedure designed to facilitate the prevention, treatment, or rehabilitation of an athletic injury. By understanding the purpose of these techniques, ATs will be better able to understand the principles and theories of athletic taping and apply them to multiple situations.

Students will learn specific taping procedures and variations of the previously described methods. They should pay close attention to how many times these basic techniques appear in the taping procedures they learn and use.

Padding, Bracing, and Protective Equipment

People involved with medieval jousting, American football, bull riding, and other sports understand how valuable padding, bracing, and protective equipment can be in preventing or lessening the severity of injuries from sporting competition. From the first chest protector, helmet, and nose guard to today's modern equipment for football and other sports, the development of protective products has become a big business. Specialized products manufactured for baseball, football, basketball, softball, soccer, lacrosse volleyball, extreme sport, outdoor activities, and other sports can fill many pages of sports medicine product catalogs.

Many types of pads, braces, and protective equipment have been developed by ATs and those interested in protecting people from injuries inherent in sport. The development of these items includes consideration of density, strength, rigidity, conformability, adherence, durability, ease of fabrication, and cost (Hillman 2005). These products have been developed in response to an observed need for protection from athletic injuries. Such equipment originally may have been conceptualized on a napkin or scrap paper before being constructed in a workshop, garage, or athletic training room. History may not reveal how some of these items have come about, except for the certainty of responding to a need for protection from harm during competition. Evolution of these items may have occurred slowly over time. Credit may never be adequately given to those involved in the development of the products, except for a patient's word of thanks or look of satisfaction following successful competition using a piece of protective equipment. For ATs, those words or glances are all the recognition needed.

As mentioned previously, there are numerous commercially developed products that meet the many padding, bracing, and equipment needs of athletes; however, in certain situations ATs might be required to manufacture their own pads out of materials available within an athletic training clinic, home, or retail store. Not all commercially available pads work for every situation, and therefore ATs must be aware of the materials, shapes, sizes, and theories available for use in their specific situation. In addition, not every employment situation provides ATs with the financial wherewithal to purchase commercially manufactured products, and they must rely on their own construction of pads or bracing. These protective items may be used alone or in combination with taping procedures and commercially available products.

The following section describes several products that are used in the development and construction of pads and braces for injury prevention during athletic activity (Beam 2006).

- Closed-cell foam
  - This foam regains its original shape quickly after deformation.
  - Provides better protection for higher levels of impact.
  - It is usually stiffer, which is less comfortable to wear.
  - Can be purchased with adhesive backing for ease of application.
- Open-cell foam
  - This foam slowly regains shape after deformation.
  - Provides better protection for low levels of impact.
  - More comfortable to wear.
  - Can be purchased with adhesive backing for ease of application.
  - Note: Pads often are manufactured using both types of foam to obtain the best of both worlds.
- Thermoldable foam
  - This closed- or open-cell foam can be heated and subsequently molded to a body part.
  - Great for padding casts and braces before competition.
- Felt
  - Varying thicknesses are available.
  - Can be used in conjunction with foams and other bracing and padding materials.

- Can be purchased with adhesive backing for ease of application.
- Gel
  - Typically made of silicone.
  - Effective in dispersing various levels of impact.
  - Comfortable to wear.
  - Can create some adherence problems.
- Heat-moldable plastics or fiberglass
  - Activated by heat or water.
  - Provides hard covering over foam or felt to increase high levels of impact.
  - Used for immobilization or range-of-motion (ROM) restriction.
- Foam or felt with hard shell
  - Soccer shin guards
  - Forearm pads
  - Hand pads
  - Pad for blocker's exostosis
- Bubble pads
  - These pads consist of a felt or foam base (next to skin) with heat-moldable plastic or plaster shell.
  - An area of foam or felt is cut out directly on top of the injured area.
  - A bump or bubble is built into the hard pad covering to facilitate force dispersion.
  - Effective for acromioclavicular joint injuries, contusions, and bursitis of the trochanter or olecranon.
- Block stop
  - Uses foam, felt, fiberglass, and other such materials to block or limit ROM.
  - Often used on the wrist, neck, elbow, and knee.
- Hinged bracing
  - Custom or off-the-shelf bracing allows functional sagittal plane movement while restricting unwanted frontal stress.
  - Most commonly used for ankle, knee, and elbow joints.

Because protective equipment for sporting activity has become a big business and there is a desire for minimal standards for maintaining competitive equality, many agencies are involved in developing and enforcing standards for equipment design and reconditioning (Hillman 2005). Many sports, conferences, leagues, and associations have minimal protective equipment requirements, and ATs must be familiar with the rules of the particular sport and level with which they are working. The minimal requirements vary depending on the league and level of play, but they are designed to protect the competitors and provide minimal guidelines and standards, eliminating unfair competitive advantage between athletes. Athletes may choose to wear additional protective equipment depending on past injury history, style of play, and personal preference, but they are not to wear less than the minimal requirements. In addition, there are also rules in place for protecting others from pads, bracing, and protective equipment that athletes are wearing. For example, participation with a cast is sometimes allowed as long as proper padding is applied to the cast to protect other participants.

ATs have a responsibility to protect their athletes, as well as those athletes their patients come in contact with. When fabricating pads, braces, or protective equipment, ATs must consult with governing agencies of the sport to see if the product conforms to the appropriate rules. In addition, care must be given to not create legal liability by creating, designing, and fabricating a pad, brace, or piece of protective equipment that will worsen an existing condition or cause an entirely new injury to athletes wearing the product or anyone they are competing against (Hillman 2005).

References

Beam, J.W. 2006. Orthopedic taping, wrapping, bracing, and padding. Philadelphia: F.A. Davis Company.

Hillman, S.K. 2005. Introduction to athletic training. Champaign, IL: Human Kinetics.

Ankle Taping, Wrapping, and Bracing

Objective

Develop and then demonstrate the ability to tape, wrap, and brace the ankle for prophylaxis or treatment of common ankle injuries.

NATA Athletic Training Educational Competencies embedded in this module: EX-C8, RM-C17, RM-C18, RM-P4, RM-P5

Competencies

1. Demonstrate the ability to apply an elastic wrap for post-ankle-sprain compression and support correctly, neatly, and quickly.

2. Demonstrate the ability to tape an ankle for prophylaxis correctly, neatly, and quickly.

3. Demonstrate the ability to tape an acutely sprained ankle correctly, neatly, and quickly so that the athlete can practice or compete.

4. Demonstrate the ability to select and apply a prophylactic ankle brace. Have the subject exercise for a few minutes to evaluate the method by which you attached the brace to the limb.

5. Demonstrate the ability to fit and apply an injury brace to an acutely sprained ankle so that an athlete can practice or compete. Have the subject exercise for a few minutes to evaluate your application.

Proficiency Demonstration

1. Develop appropriate subject knowledge through coursework (C), verbal conversation (V), quizzes (Q), worksheets (W), or other approved activities (O).

2. Practice and reinforce the skills in clinical skills and laboratory courses.

3. Refine your skills by observing peer teachers and clinical instructors as they perform the skills (preferably on patients), discussing the competencies with peer teachers and clinical instructors, practicing alone and with others, and then demonstrating proficiency to a peer teacher.

4. Demonstrate your proficiency to an ACI.

APPROVED BY
(date and signature, and mode for didactic)

1. Elastic wrap

Didactic _____

Lab _____

Peer _____

ACI _____

2. Prophylactic tape

Didactic _____

Lab _____

Peer _____

ACI _____

3. Injury tape

Didactic _____

Lab _____

Peer _____

ACI _____

4. Prophylactic brace

Didactic _____

Lab _____

Peer _____

ACI _____

5. Injury brace

Didactic _____

Lab _____

Peer _____

ACI _____

COMMENTS

_____

_____

_____

_____

_____

_____

_____

Knee Taping, Wrapping, and Bracing

Objective

Develop and then demonstrate the ability to tape, wrap, and brace the knee for prophylaxis or treatment of common knee injuries.

NATA Athletic Training Educational Competencies embedded in this module: EX-C8, RM-C17, RM-C18, RM-P4, RM-P5

Competencies

1. Demonstrate the ability to apply elastic wraps correctly, neatly, and quickly for immediate care of the following conditions:

    a. Collateral ligament sprain
    b. Hyperextension sprain

2. Demonstrate the ability to correctly, neatly, and quickly tape the knee to allow the athlete to practice or compete during the latter phases of rehabilitation of the following injuries:

    a. Medial collateral knee ligament (medial and lateral)
    b. Hyperextended knee
    c. Patellofemoral pain

3. Discuss the differences and similarities in the design and use of various types and brands of knee braces.

4. Demonstrate the ability to select and apply the following knee braces. Have the subject exercise for a few minutes to evaluate the method by which you attached the brace to the limb.

    a. Prophylactic brace
    b. Postinjury or postsurgery immobilization brace
    c. Medial collateral ligament (MCL) or lateral collateral ligament (LCL) brace
    d. Anterior cruciate ligament (ACL) or posterior cruciate ligament (PCL) brace
    e. Patellar tracking brace

Proficiency Demonstration

1. Develop appropriate subject knowledge through coursework (C), verbal conversation (V), quizzes (Q), worksheets (W), or other approved activities (O).

2. Practice and reinforce the skills in clinical skills and laboratory courses.

3. Refine your skills by observing peer teachers and clinical instructors as they perform the skills (preferably on patients), discussing the competencies with peer teachers and clinical instructors, practicing alone and with others, and then demonstrating proficiency to a peer teacher.

4. Demonstrate your proficiency to an ACI.

APPROVED BY
(date and signature, and mode for didactic)

1a. Elastic wrap—collateral ligament sprain

    Didactic _____

    Lab _____

    Peer _____

    ACI _____

1b. Elastic wrap—hyperextension sprain

    Didactic _____

    Lab _____

    Peer _____

    ACI _____

2a. Tape—medial collateral knee ligament

    Didactic _____

    Lab _____

    Peer _____

    ACI _____

2b. Tape—hyperextended knee

    Didactic _____

    Lab _____

    Peer _____

    ACI _____

2c. Tape—patellofemoral pain

    Didactic _____

    Lab _____

    Peer _____

    ACI _____

3. Knee brace discussion

    Didactic _____

    Lab _____

    Peer _____

    ACI _____

4a. Prophylactic brace

Didactic _____

Lab _____

Peer _____

ACI _____

4b. Injury immobilizer

Didactic _____

Lab _____

Peer _____

ACI _____

4c. MCL or LCL brace

Didactic _____

Lab _____

Peer _____

ACI _____

4d. ACL or PCL brace

Didactic _____

Lab _____

Peer _____

ACI _____

4e. Patellar brace

Didactic _____

Lab _____

Peer _____

ACI _____

COMMENTS

_____

_____

_____

_____

_____

_____

_____

Thigh and Lower-Leg Taping, Wrapping, and Padding

Objective

Develop and then demonstrate the ability to tape, wrap, and pad the thigh and lower leg for prophylaxis or treatment of common injuries of the thigh and lower leg.

NATA Athletic Training Educational Competencies embedded in this module: EX-C8, RM-C17, RM-C18, RM-P4, RM-P5

Competencies

1. Demonstrate the ability to apply elastic wraps correctly, neatly, and quickly for immediate care of a thigh strain.

2. Demonstrate the ability to correctly, neatly, and quickly tape the lower leg to allow the athlete to practice or compete during the latter phases of rehabilitation of the following injuries:

    a. Achilles tendon strain
    b. Medial tibial stress syndrome

3. Discuss the types of material used to construct injury pads and show how each is used.

4. Fabricate a heat-moldable pad.

5. Demonstrate the ability to select and apply pads for the following injuries. Have the subject exercise for a few minutes to evaluate the method by which you attached the pad.

    a. Quadriceps contusion
    b. Shin contusion

Proficiency Demonstration

1. Develop appropriate subject knowledge through coursework (C), verbal conversation (V), quizzes (Q), worksheets (W), or other approved activities (O).

2. Practice and reinforce the skills in clinical skills and laboratory courses.

3. Refine your skills by observing peer teachers and clinical instructors as they perform the skills (preferably on patients), discussing the competencies with peer teachers and clinical instructors, practicing alone and with others, and then demonstrating proficiency to a peer teacher.

4. Demonstrate your proficiency to an ACI.

APPROVED BY
(date and signature, and mode for didactic)

1. Elastic wrap

    Didactic _____

    Lab _____

    Peer _____

    ACI _____

2a. Tape—Achilles tendon strain

    Didactic _____

    Lab _____

    Peer _____

    ACI _____

2b. Tape—medial tibial stress syndrome

    Didactic _____

    Lab _____

    Peer _____

    ACI _____

3. Discussion of pad materials

    Didactic _____

    Lab _____

    Peer _____

    ACI _____

4. Heat-moldable pad fabrication

    Didactic _____

    Lab _____

    Peer _____

    ACI _____

5a. Pad—quadriceps contusion

    Didactic _____

    Lab _____

    Peer _____

    ACI _____

5b. Pad—shin contusion

Didactic _____

Lab _____

Peer _____

ACI _____

COMMENTS

_____

_____

_____

Foot Care, Taping, Wrapping, and Padding

Objective

Develop and then demonstrate the ability to care for, tape, wrap, and pad the foot for prophylaxis or treatment of common foot injuries and conditions.

NATA Athletic Training Educational Competencies embedded in this module: EX-C8, RM-C17, RM-C18, RM-P4, RM-P5

Competencies

1. Demonstrate the ability to care for the following foot injuries:

    a. Blisters
    b. Corns and bunions
    c. Ingrown toenails

2. Demonstrate the ability to correctly, neatly, and quickly tape the foot to allow the athlete to practice or compete during the latter phases of rehabilitation of the following injuries:

    a. Sprained hallux
    b. Sprained digit
    c. Longitudinal arch
    d. Heel bruise

3. Discuss the differences and similarities in the design and use of various types and brands of specialty foot pads.

4. Demonstrate the ability to select and apply the following foot pads. Have the subject exercise for a few minutes to evaluate the method by which you attached the pad to the limb.

    a. Metatarsal stress fracture
    b. Toe fracture
    c. Heel spur
    d. Heel bruise

Proficiency Demonstration

1. Develop appropriate subject knowledge through coursework (C), verbal conversation (V), quizzes (Q), worksheets (W), or other approved activities (O).

2. Practice and reinforce the skills in clinical skills and laboratory courses.

3. Refine your skills by observing peer teachers and clinical instructors as they perform the skills (preferably on patients), discussing the competencies with peer teachers and clinical instructors, practicing alone and with others, and then demonstrating proficiency to a peer teacher.

4. Demonstrate your proficiency to an ACI.

APPROVED BY
(date and signature, and mode for didactic)

1a. Care—blisters

    Didactic _____

    Lab _____

    Peer _____

    ACI _____

1b. Care—corns and bunions

    Didactic _____

    Lab _____

    Peer _____

    ACI _____

1c. Care—ingrown toenails

    Didactic _____

    Lab _____

    Peer _____

    ACI _____

2a. Tape—sprained hallux

    Didactic _____

    Lab _____

    Peer _____

    ACI _____

2b. Tape—sprained digit

    Didactic _____

    Lab _____

    Peer _____

    ACI _____

2c. Tape—longitudinal arch

    Didactic _____

    Lab _____

    Peer _____

    ACI _____

2d. Tape—heel bruise

    Didactic _____

    Lab _____

Peer _____

ACI _____

3. Discussion of specialty foot pads

Didactic _____

Lab _____

Peer _____

ACI _____

4a. Pad—metatarsal stress fracture

Didactic _____

Lab _____

Peer _____

ACI _____

4b. Pad—toe fracture

Didactic _____

Lab _____

Peer _____

ACI _____

4c. Pad—heel spur

Didactic _____

Lab _____

Peer _____

ACI _____

4d. Pad—heel bruise

Didactic _____

Lab _____

Peer _____

ACI _____

COMMENTS

_____

_____

_____

_____

Hip and Abdomen Taping, Wrapping, and Bracing

Objective

Develop and then demonstrate the ability to tape and wrap the hip and abdomen for prophylaxis or treatment of common hip and abdomen injuries.

NATA Athletic Training Educational Competencies embedded in this module: EX-C8, RM-C17, RM-C18, RM-P4, RM-P5

Competencies

1. Demonstrate the ability to apply elastic wraps correctly, neatly, and quickly for immediate care of the following two conditions:

    a. Hip strain—adductors

    b. Hip strain—flexors

2. Demonstrate the ability to correctly, neatly, and quickly tape the hip and abdomen to allow the athlete to practice or compete during the latter phases of rehabilitation of a hip pointer.

3. Demonstrate the ability to select and apply a brace for a lumbosacral sprain. Have the subject exercise for a few minutes to evaluate the method by which you attached the brace to the limb.

Proficiency Demonstration

1. Develop appropriate subject knowledge through coursework (C), verbal conversation (V), quizzes (Q), worksheets (W), or other approved activities (O).

2. Practice and reinforce the skills in clinical skills and laboratory courses.

3. Refine your skills by observing peer teachers and clinical instructors as they perform the skills (preferably on patients), discussing the competencies with peer teachers and clinical instructors, practicing alone and with others, and then demonstrating proficiency to a peer teacher.

4. Demonstrate your proficiency to an ACI.

APPROVED BY
(date and signature, and mode for didactic)

1a. Hip strain—adductors

Didactic _____

Lab _____

Peer _____

ACI _____

1b. Hip strain—flexors

Didactic _____

Lab _____

Peer _____

ACI _____

2. Hip pointer

Didactic _____

Lab _____

Peer _____

ACI _____

3. Lumbosacral sprain

Didactic _____

Lab _____

Peer _____

ACI _____

COMMENTS

_____

_____

_____

Shoulder Taping, Wrapping, and Bracing

Objective

Develop and then demonstrate the ability to tape, wrap, and brace the shoulder for prophylaxis or treatment of common shoulder injuries.

Competencies

1. Demonstrate the ability to apply the following bandages to the shoulder correctly, neatly, and quickly for immediate care of a shoulder injury:

    a. Shoulder sling (cloth)
    b. Shoulder sling (elastic wraps)
    c. Shoulder spica (elastic wraps)

2. Demonstrate the ability to correctly, neatly, and quickly tape the shoulder and chest to allow the athlete to practice or compete during the latter phases of rehabilitation of the following:

    a. Acromioclavicular sprain
    b. Sternoclavicular sprain

3. Discuss the differences and similarities in the design and use of various types and brands of shoulder braces.

4. Demonstrate the ability to select and apply the following shoulder pads and braces. Have the subject exercise for a few minutes to evaluate the method by which you attached the brace to the limb.

    a. Shoulder harness
    b. Shoulder pads
    c. Acromioclavicular pad
    d. Sternoclavicular pad

Proficiency Demonstration

1. Develop appropriate subject knowledge through coursework (C), verbal conversation (V), quizzes (Q), worksheets (W), or other approved activities (O).

2. Practice and reinforce the skills in clinical skills and laboratory courses.

3. Refine your skills by observing peer teachers and clinical instructors as they perform the skills (preferably on patients), discussing the competencies with peer teachers and clinical instructors, practicing alone and with others, and then demonstrating proficiency to a peer teacher.

4. Demonstrate your proficiency to an ACI.

APPROVED BY
(date and signature, and mode for didactic)

1a. Sling—cloth
    Didactic _____
    Lab _____
    Peer _____
    ACI _____

1b. Sling—elastic
    Didactic _____
    Lab _____
    Peer _____
    ACI _____

1c. Shoulder spica
    Didactic _____
    Lab _____
    Peer _____
    ACI _____

2a. Acromioclavicular tape
    Didactic _____
    Lab _____
    Peer _____
    ACI _____

2b. Sternoclavicular tape
    Didactic _____
    Lab _____
    Peer _____
    ACI _____

3. Discussion of shoulder braces
    Didactic _____
    Lab _____
    Peer _____
    ACI _____

4a. Shoulder harness

Didactic _____

Lab _____

Peer _____

ACI _____

4b. Shoulder pads

Didactic _____

Lab _____

Peer _____

ACI _____

4c. Acromioclavicular pad

Didactic _____

Lab _____

Peer _____

ACI _____

4d. Sternoclavicular pad

Didactic _____

Lab _____

Peer _____

ACI _____

COMMENTS

_____

_____

_____

_____

_____

_____

Elbow-to-Wrist Taping, Wrapping, and Bracing

Objective

Develop and then demonstrate the ability to tape, wrap, and brace the elbow, forearm, and wrist for prophylaxis or treatment of common elbow, forearm, and wrist injuries.

NATA Athletic Training Educational Competencies embedded in this module: EX-C8, RM-C17, RM-C18, RM-P4, RM-P5

Competencies

1. Demonstrate the ability to apply elastic wraps correctly, neatly, and quickly for immediate care of an elbow contusion.

2. Demonstrate the ability to apply elastic or cloth wraps to the wrist correctly, neatly, and quickly to allow an athlete with a sprained wrist to practice or compete during the latter phases of rehabilitation in the following two sports:

    a. American football
    b. Gymnastics

3. Demonstrate the ability to apply a double-friction blister pad to the wrist of a gymnast with severe blisters to allow the athlete to compete on rings or bars.

4. Demonstrate the ability to correctly, neatly, and quickly tape the elbow, arm, and wrist to allow the athlete to practice or compete during the latter phases of rehabilitation of the following injuries:

    a. Elbow hyperextension
    b. Collateral ligament sprain
    c. Forearm splints
    d. Wrist flexor strain
    e. Wrist extensor strain

5. Discuss the differences and similarities in the design and use of various types and brands of elbow braces.

6. Demonstrate the ability to select and apply the following brace and pad. Have the subject exercise for a few minutes to evaluate the method by which you attached the brace to the limb.

    a. Epicondylitis
    b. Olecranon bursa contusion using closed-cell foam

Proficiency Demonstration

1. Develop appropriate subject knowledge through coursework (C), verbal conversation (V), quizzes (Q), worksheets (W), or other approved activities (O).

2. Practice and reinforce the skills in clinical skills and laboratory courses.

3. Refine your skills by observing peer teachers and clinical instructors as they perform the skills (preferably on patients), discussing the competencies with peer teachers and clinical instructors, practicing alone and with others, and then demonstrating proficiency to a peer teacher.

4. Demonstrate your proficiency to an ACI.

APPROVED BY
(date and signature, and mode for didactic)

  1. Elbow contusion

    Didactic _____

    Lab _____

    Peer _____

    ACI _____

 2a. Sprained wrist—football

    Didactic _____

    Lab _____

    Peer _____

    ACI _____

 2b. Sprained wrist—gymnastics

    Didactic _____

    Lab _____

    Peer _____

    ACI _____

  3. Wrist—friction blister

    Didactic _____

    Lab _____

    Peer _____

    ACI _____

4a. Elbow hyperextension

Didactic _____

Lab _____

Peer _____

ACI _____

4b. Collateral ligament sprain

Didactic _____

Lab _____

Peer _____

ACI _____

4c. Forearm splints

Didactic _____

Lab _____

Peer _____

ACI _____

4d. Wrist flexor strain

Didactic _____

Lab _____

Peer _____

ACI _____

4e. Wrist extensor sprain

Didactic _____

Lab _____

Peer _____

ACI _____

5. Elbow braces discussion

Didactic _____

Lab _____

Peer _____

ACI _____

6a. Epicondylitis

Didactic _____

Lab _____

Peer _____

ACI _____

6b. Olecranon bursa contusion

Didactic _____

Lab _____

Peer _____

ACI _____

COMMENTS

_____

_____

_____

_____

_____

Hand and Finger Taping and Wrapping

Objective

Develop and then demonstrate the ability to tape and wrap the hand and fingers for prophylaxis or treatment of common hand and finger injuries.

NATA Athletic Training Educational Competencies embedded in this module: EX-C8, RM-C17, RM-C18, RM-P4, RM-P5

Competencies

1. Demonstrate the ability to tape a sprained finger correctly, neatly, and quickly as part of immediate care.

2. Demonstrate the ability to correctly, neatly, and quickly tape the hand and fingers to allow the athlete to practice or compete during the latter phases of rehabilitation of the following injuries:

   a. Hand contusion
   b. Thumb sprain
   c. Proximal interphalangeal (PIP) sprain
   d. Distal interphalangeal (DIP) sprain
   e. Boutonniere
   f. Finger dislocation
   g. Finger hyperextension
   h. Mallet finger

Proficiency Demonstration

1. Develop appropriate subject knowledge through coursework (C), verbal conversation (V), quizzes (Q), worksheets (W), or other approved activities (O).

2. Practice and reinforce the skills in clinical skills and laboratory courses.

3. Refine your skills by observing peer teachers and clinical instructors as they perform the skills (preferably on patients), discussing the competencies with peer teachers and clinical instructors, practicing alone and with others, and then demonstrating proficiency to a peer teacher.

4. Demonstrate your proficiency to an ACI.

APPROVED BY
(date and signature, and mode for didactic)

1. Finger sprain
   Didactic _____
   Lab _____
   Peer _____
   ACI _____

2a. Hand contusion
   Didactic _____
   Lab _____
   Peer _____
   ACI _____

2b. Thumb sprain
   Didactic _____
   Lab _____
   Peer _____
   ACI _____

2c. PIP sprain
   Didactic _____
   Lab _____
   Peer _____
   ACI _____

2d. DIP sprain
   Didactic _____
   Lab _____
   Peer _____
   ACI _____

2e. Boutonniere
   Didactic _____
   Lab _____
   Peer _____
   ACI _____

2f. Finger dislocation
   Didactic _____
   Lab _____
   Peer _____
   ACI _____

2g. Finger hyperextension
   Didactic _____
   Lab _____
   Peer _____
   ACI _____

2h. Mallet finger

Didactic _____

Lab _____

Peer _____

ACI _____

COMMENTS

_____

_____

_____

Head and Neck Padding and Bracing

Objective

Develop and then demonstrate the ability to pad and brace the head and neck for prophylaxis or treatment of common head and neck injuries.

NATA Athletic Training Educational Competencies embedded in this module: EX-C8, RM-C17, RM-C18, RM-P4, RM-P5

Competencies

1. Fit an off-the-shelf mouthpiece or manufacture a custom mouthpiece (the type used by your athletic department).

2. Manufacture or fit a customized face mask to a basketball player to protect a facial or nose fracture.

3. Fit a neck roll to prevent a neck hyperextension injury.

4. Fit a cervical collar for emergency management of a neck injury.

Proficiency Demonstration

1. Develop appropriate subject knowledge through coursework (C), verbal conversation (V), quizzes (Q), worksheets (W), or other approved activities (O).

2. Practice and reinforce the skills in clinical skills and laboratory courses.

3. Refine your skills by observing peer teachers and clinical instructors as they perform the skills (preferably on patients), discussing the competencies with peer teachers and clinical instructors, practicing alone and with others, and then demonstrating proficiency to a peer teacher.

4. Demonstrate your proficiency to an ACI.

APPROVED BY
(date and signature, and mode for didactic)

1. Mouthpiece

Didactic _____

Lab _____

Peer _____

ACI _____

2. Face mask

Didactic _____

Lab _____

Peer _____

ACI _____

3. Neck roll

Didactic _____

Lab _____

Peer _____

ACI _____

4. Collar

Didactic _____

Lab _____

Peer _____

ACI _____

COMMENTS

_____

_____

_____

Level 2.6

Risk Management

Prevention of injuries caused by physical activity is one of the practice domains for ATs. It is an area that has ramifications for many people, including the athlete, coach, team, and health care community. By working to prevent injuries, the AT helps the athlete decrease or eliminate participation time loss due to injury. If the person is a member of a team, this injury prevention has the ability to make a difference in the enjoyment and success of competitive events or seasons. In addition, prevention of athletic injuries has a beneficial impact on the health care system by lessening the burden on health care personnel, facilities, and insurance.

Risk management, a component of prevention, applies to all ATs, and it should be a critical injury prevention consideration during the precompetitive time, as well as in the day-to-day contact between the AT and the athletes. Risk management is an administrative function directed toward identification, evaluation, and correction of risks that could lead to injury to patients, staff members, or others.

Evaluation of anthropometric measurements and other physical screening measurements provides important information regarding the physical ability for healthy participation. Abnormalities or out-of-normal-range measurements should be addressed by appropriate medical practitioners. Other aspects of risk management practices encompass facility and equipment considerations. Protective equipment for safe participation must be obtained, maintained, and fitted. Facilities must be designed, constructed, and maintained to allow appropriate and safe competition. Instruction in and planning of individual and team programs for improvement of flexibility, strength, and cardiorespiratory conditioning based on anthropometric measurements, physical screenings, and sport-specific demands also helps lessen the risks that could lead to injury to athletes.

The modules in this section allow students to explore, examine, and apply individual skill sets that fall under the auspices of risk management. Prevention of athletic injuries occurs via the following activities:

Screening

Personal protective equipment

Recognition of risk factors

Strength and conditioning

Flexibility

Proper and well-maintained equipment

Facility management

Emergency care

Taping, bracing, wrapping, and padding

Policies and procedures

Environmental injuries and illnesses

Time limits

Anthropometric Measurements and Screening Procedures

Objective

Develop the skills necessary to perform anthropometric measurements and other appropriate examination and screening procedures.

NATA Athletic Training Educational Competencies embedded in this module: DI-P5, RM-C3, RM-C4, RM-C5, RM-C11, NU-C18, NU-P1

Competencies

1. Use reliable sources for epidemiological data regarding injuries and illnesses to facilitate concept development and performance of wellness screening.

2. Identify known physical and physiological demands and risks associated with various athletic activities. Discuss components of preparticipation screening and examinations to reduce these risks. At a minimum, they should include the following:
   a. Cardiorespiratory fitness
   b. Respiratory fitness
   c. Muscular strength, power, and endurance
   d. Flexibility
   e. Posture and gait
   f. Body composition

3. Define *measurement reliability* and *measurement validity* and discuss how each relates to anthropometric measurements and screening procedures.

4. Measure the following on at least five people on two different days (10 people total). Record your results.
   a. Height
   b. Weight
   c. Blood pressure
   d. Pulse
   e. Limb girth
   f. Limb length
   g. Passive ROM (using a goniometer)
   h. Active ROM (using a goniometer)
   i. Vision (using a Snellen eye chart)
   j. Body composition (using a manual skinfold caliper and appropriate formulas)

5. Discuss the results of the measurements in competency 2, including how they relate to measurement reliability and validity.

Proficiency Demonstration

1. Develop appropriate subject knowledge through coursework (C), verbal conversation (V), quizzes (Q), worksheets (W), or other approved activities (O).

2. Practice and reinforce the skills in clinical skills and laboratory courses.

3. Refine your skills by observing peer teachers and clinical instructors as they perform the skills (preferably on patients), discussing the competencies with peer teachers and clinical instructors, practicing alone and with others, and then demonstrating proficiency to a peer teacher.

4. Demonstrate your proficiency to an ACI.

APPROVED BY
(date and signature, and mode for didactic)

1. Epidemiological data for concept development
   Didactic _____
   Lab _____
   Peer _____
   ACI _____

2. Preparticipation exam discussion
   Didactic _____
   Lab _____
   Peer _____
   ACI _____

3. Reliability and validity definition
   Didactic _____
   Lab _____
   Peer _____
   ACI _____

4. Measurements
   Didactic _____
   Lab _____
   Peer _____
   ACI _____

5. Discussion of measurement reliability and validity
   Didactic _____
   Lab _____
   Peer _____
   ACI _____

COMMENTS
_____

_____

Protective Equipment Fitting

Objective

Develop and demonstrate the skills necessary to select, fit, modify, and create protective athletic equipment.

NATA Athletic Training Educational Competencies embedded in this module: EX-C8, RM-C16, RM-P4, RM-CP2

Competencies

1. Access information about the regulations and standards for the use of protective equipment in sport. Use sport rule books, textbooks, information resources, and the listed Web sites to do the following:

   a. Explain the mission and basic principles of equipment regulatory agencies and associations.

   b. Determine the agency responsible for standards associated with helmet use for American football, lacrosse, ice hockey, baseball, and softball.

   c. Create a list of 10 facts you did not know about the manufacturing, certification, reconditioning, and recertification of protective sport equipment.

      www.ncaa.org
      www.nfhs.org
      www.nata.org
      http://naia.org

2. Select and fit the following protective equipment to at least two athletes:

   a. Protective helmet and head gear for football, ice hockey, and lacrosse

   b. Football and hockey shoulder pads

   c. Footwear for physical activity

   d. Rib brace or guard

   e. Mouth guard

   f. Knee brace (ACL, MCL, patellofemoral)

   g. Ankle brace (lace up, strap, double upright)

   h. Neck collars, rolls, and plates

   i. Miscellaneous hand, wrist, elbow, shoulder, knee, back, hip, and lower-leg pads, braces, and splints

3. Create or modify an existing pad using additional foam, felt, or thermoplastic material to protect patients who have suffered the following:

   a. Hip pointer

   b. Acromioclavicular joint sprain

   c. Olecranon or prepatellar bursitis

Proficiency Demonstration

1. Develop appropriate subject knowledge through coursework (C), verbal conversation (V), quizzes (Q), worksheets (W), or other approved activities (O).

2. Practice and reinforce the skills in clinical skills and laboratory courses.

3. Refine your skills by observing peer teachers and clinical instructors as they perform the skills (preferably on patients), discussing the competencies with peer teachers and clinical instructors, practicing alone and with others, and then demonstrating proficiency to a peer teacher.

4. Demonstrate your proficiency to an ACI.

APPROVED BY
(date and signature, and mode for didactic)

1. Protective equipment standards and regulations

   Didactic _____

   Lab _____

   Peer _____

   ACI _____

2. Protective equipment selection and fit

   Didactic _____

   Lab _____

   Peer _____

   ACI _____

3. Creation or modification of existing pad

   Didactic _____

   Lab _____

   Peer _____

   ACI _____

COMMENTS

_____

_____

_____

_____

Ergonomics and Injury Prevention

Objective

Develop an understanding of the role that work, home, school, lifting, and activity ergonomics play in the prevention of injuries.

NATA Athletic Training Educational Competencies embedded in this module: RM-C19, RM-P3

Competencies

1. Describe ergonomics as if you were explaining it to someone not associated with the health profession.

2. Discuss injuries that are typically associated with improper ergonomics, such as poor posture, improper lifting techniques, repetitive movements, extreme force, and overuse.

3. Describe the benefits of proper ergonomics.

4. Discuss ways to improve the ergonomics of various daily activities both in your clinic and outside of it.

5. Demonstrate ergonomic positions for lifting, sitting, rising from prone or supine positions, standing, and other activities of daily living.

Proficiency Demonstration

1. Develop appropriate subject knowledge through coursework (C), verbal conversation (V), quizzes (Q), worksheets (W), or other approved activities (O).

2. Practice and reinforce the skills in clinical skills and laboratory courses.

3. Refine your skills by observing peer teachers and clinical instructors as they perform the skills (preferably on patients), discussing the competencies with peer teachers and clinical instructors, practicing alone and with others, and then demonstrating proficiency to a peer teacher.

4. Demonstrate your proficiency to an ACI.

APPROVED BY
(date and signature, and mode for didactic)

1. Description of ergonomics

Didactic _____

Lab _____

Peer _____

ACI _____

2. Improper ergonomics

Didactic _____

Lab _____

Peer _____

ACI _____

3. Proper ergonomics

Didactic _____

Lab _____

Peer _____

ACI _____

4. Ergonomic improvement

Didactic _____

Lab _____

Peer _____

ACI _____

5. Ergonomic demonstration

Didactic _____

Lab _____

Peer _____

ACI _____

COMMENTS

_____

_____

_____

_____

_____

_____

Fitness Testing

Objective

Understand the principles and application of various fitness assessment tests.

NATA Athletic Training Educational Competencies embedded in this module: RM-C11, RM-P1

Competencies

1. Describe the rationale for testing the following components of fitness:
  a. Strength
  b. Power
  c. Muscular endurance
  d. Speed
  e. Balance
  f. Agility
  g. Flexibility
  h. Cardiorespiratory endurance
  i. Posture and gait
  j. Body composition

2. Describe and demonstrate two tests and their procedures for evaluating each of the elements in competency 1.

Proficiency Demonstration

1. Develop appropriate subject knowledge through coursework (C), verbal conversation (V), quizzes (Q), worksheets (W), or other approved activities (O).

2. Practice and reinforce the skills in clinical skills and laboratory courses.

3. Refine your skills by observing peer teachers and clinical instructors as they perform the skills (preferably on patients), discussing the competencies with peer teachers and clinical instructors, practicing alone and with others, and then demonstrating proficiency to a peer teacher.

4. Demonstrate your proficiency to an ACI.

APPROVED BY
(date and signature, and mode for didactic)

1. Rationale for fitness tests

Didactic _____

Lab _____

Peer _____

ACI _____

2. Tests and procedures

Didactic _____

Lab _____

Peer _____

ACI _____

COMMENTS

_____

_____

_____

_____

_____

_____

_____

Flimbility Training

Objective

Develop and demonstrate the skills necessary to develop flexibility.

NATA Athletic Training Educational Competencies embedded in this module: RM-C11, RM-C13, RM-P1, RM-P2

Competencies

Instruct and demonstrate exercises to develop flexibility for the following:

- **a.** Cervical region
- **b.** Shoulder girdle
- **c.** Elbow
- **d.** Wrist
- **e.** Hand and fingers
- **f.** Lumbar region
- **g.** Hip and pelvis
- **h.** Knee
- **i.** Lower leg
- **j.** Ankle
- **k.** Foot and toes

Proficiency Demonstration

1. Develop appropriate subject knowledge through coursework (C), verbal conversation (V), quizzes (Q), worksheets (W), or other approved activities (O).

2. Practice and reinforce the skills in clinical skills and laboratory courses.

3. Refine your skills by observing peer teachers and clinical instructors as they perform the skills (preferably on patients), discussing the competencies with peer teachers and clinical instructors, practicing alone and with others, and then demonstrating proficiency to a peer teacher.

4. Demonstrate your proficiency to an ACI.

APPROVED BY
(date and signature, and mode for didactic)

1a. Cervical region

Didactic _____

Lab _____

Peer _____

ACI _____

1b. Shoulder girdle

Didactic _____

Lab _____

Peer _____

ACI _____

1c. Elbow

Didactic _____

Lab _____

Peer _____

ACI _____

1d. Wrist

Didactic _____

Lab _____

Peer _____

ACI _____

1e. Hand and fingers

Didactic _____

Lab _____

Peer _____

ACI _____

1f. Lumbar region

Didactic _____

Lab _____

Peer _____

ACI _____

1g. Hip and pelvis

Didactic _____

Lab _____

Peer _____

ACI _____

1h. Knee

Didactic _____

Lab _____

Peer _____

ACI _____

1i. Lower leg

Didactic _____

Lab _____

Peer _____

ACI _____

1j. Ankle

Didactic _____

Lab _____

Peer _____

ACI _____

1k. Foot and toes

Didactic _____

Lab _____

Peer _____

ACI _____

COMMENTS

_____

_____

Strength Training

Objective

Develop and demonstrate the skills necessary to teach strength training techniques.

NATA Athletic Training Educational Competencies embedded in this module: RM-C1, RM-P1, RM-P3, EX-C2, EX-P4, EX-P5

Competencies

1. Instruct and demonstrate lifting technique for the following. Point out common dangerous or unsafe techniques.

    a. Parallel squat
    b. Heel raise
    c. Power clean
    d. Bench press
    e. Shoulder press
    f. Deadlift
    g. Arm curl
    h. Triceps extension
    i. Knee curl (flexion)
    j. Knee extension
    k. Leg press

2. Instruct and demonstrate spotting technique for the following:

    a. Parallel squat
    b. Shoulder press
    c. Deadlift
    d. Bench press
    e. Power clean

Proficiency Demonstration

1. Develop appropriate subject knowledge through coursework (C), verbal conversation (V), quizzes (Q), worksheets (W), or other approved activities (O).

2. Practice and reinforce the skills in clinical skills and laboratory courses.

3. Refine your skills by observing peer teachers and clinical instructors as they perform the skills (preferably on patients), discussing the competencies with peer teachers and clinical instructors, practicing alone and with others, and then demonstrating proficiency to a peer teacher.

4. Demonstrate your proficiency to an ACI.

APPROVED BY
(date and signature, and mode for didactic)

1a. Parallel squat

Didactic _____

Lab _____

Peer _____

ACI _____

1b. Heel raise

Didactic _____

Lab _____

Peer _____

ACI _____

1c. Power clean

Didactic _____

Lab _____

Peer _____

ACI _____

1d. Bench press

Didactic _____

Lab _____

Peer _____

ACI _____

1e. Shoulder press

Didactic _____

Lab _____

Peer _____

ACI _____

1f. Deadlift

Didactic _____

Lab _____

Peer _____

ACI _____

1g. Arm curl

Didactic _____

Lab _____

Peer _____

ACI _____

1h. Triceps extension

Didactic _____

Lab _____

Peer _____

ACI _____

1i. Knee curl (flexion)

Didactic _____

Lab _____

Peer _____

ACI _____

1j. Knee extension

Didactic _____

Lab _____

Peer _____

ACI _____

1k. Leg press

Didactic _____

Lab _____

Peer _____

ACI _____

2a. Spotting—parallel squat

Didactic _____

Lab _____

Peer _____

ACI _____

2b. Spotting—shoulder press

Didactic _____

Lab _____

Peer _____

ACI _____

2c. Spotting—deadlift

Didactic _____

Lab _____

Peer _____

ACI _____

2d. Spotting—bench press

Didactic _____

Lab _____

Peer _____

ACI _____

2e. Spotting—power clean

Didactic _____

Lab _____

Peer _____

ACI _____

COMMENTS

_____

_____

_____

_____

_____

Level 2.7

Basic Nutrition, Pharmacology, and Wellness

Understanding the application and regulations of pharmacology within the practice of athletic training is an important component of patient care. ATs must understand pharmacology use, misuse, and abuse during emergency response, injury and illness prevention, treatment, rehabilitation, and performance enhancement. Knowledge of pharmacological applications and the ability to acquire additional information in this subject area is critical to continued care and treatment of patients.

In addition, familiarity with the effects of basic nutrition upon the athlete can facilitate physical performance and recovery. Helping others maintain a healthy lifestyle and enhance their performance through proper nutritional habits is a fundamental component of prevention, treatment, and recovery of athletic injuries and illnesses. It is important for ATs to understand current governmental guidelines and be aware of information sources they can use in guiding others toward healthy eating in order to meet the energy demands placed on the body during training, competition, and rehabilitation.

Athletic training students will not be asked to learn all there is to know about pharmacology and nutrition; that is beyond the scope of the module series. However, it is important for students to develop a working understanding of how pharmacology and nutrition affect the prevention, treatment, and recovery process of injuries, illnesses, and disease found among their patient populations. The following modules will guide the students as they review common prescription and nonprescription medications, become familiar with medical terminology and abbreviations associated with pharmacology, understand the processes of pharmacodynamics and pharmacokinetics, describe administration procedures, explain manufacturing and marketing influence, outline medication treatment protocols, summarize the drug-approval process of the national governing agency (e.g., U.S. Food and Drug Administration [FDA]), follow poison control protocols, identify information resources, clarify athletes' misperceptions regarding performance-enhancing substances, differentiate among major drug classifications, understand the role of nutrition for the competing athlete, identify common eating disorders, and become an authoritative source of information regarding pharmacology and nutrition for their patients.

Medication Resources

Objective

Develop and demonstrate the skills necessary to use the *Physician's Desk Reference (PDR), Drug Facts and Comparisons,* or online resources for obtaining information on medications related to athletic training.

NATA Athletic Training Educational Competencies embedded in this module: PH-C2, PH-C3, PH-C7, PH-C8, PH-P1

Competencies

Use the *PDR* or another drug reference to search for information on medications commonly prescribed to people involved in physical activity and to identify the following information:

a. Generic and brand names

b. Indications for use

c. Contraindications

d. Warnings

e. Dosage

f. Other notes (e.g., banned substance)

g. Side (adverse) effects

Proficiency Demonstration

1. Develop appropriate subject knowledge through coursework (C), verbal conversation (V), quizzes (Q), worksheets (W), or other approved activities (O).

2. Refine your knowledge through discussions with peer teachers and clinical instructors.

3. Demonstrate proficiency to a peer teacher and an ACI.

APPROVED BY
(date and signature, and mode for didactic)

Medication resource
Didactic _____

Peer _____

ACI _____

COMMENTS

_____

_____

_____

_____

_____

_____

Medication Physiology

Objective

Demonstrate an understanding of the physiological processes involved with medication use.

NATA Athletic Training Educational Competencies imbedded in this module: PH-C4, PH-C5, PH-C6, PH-C7

Competencies

1. Discuss the following concepts as they relate to the biochemistry and physiology of pharmaceuticals.

    a. pharmacokinetics
    b. pharmacodynamics
    c. absorption
    d. distribution
    e. metabolism
    f. elimination
    g. bioavailability
    h. half-life
    i. bioequivalence

2. Discuss the following terms and concepts as they relate to pharmacodynamics:

    a. drug action
    b. therapeutic effectiveness
    c. receptor theory
    d. dose-response relationship
    e. potency
    f. drug interactions

3. Discuss the influence that exercise has on each of the concepts in #1 (as related to pharmaceuticals).

4. Discuss the process, advantages, and disadvantages of the following modes of administering medications:

    a. oral
    b. inhalation
    c. injection
    d. iontophoresis
    e. phonophoresis

Proficiency Demonstration

1. Develop appropriate subject knowledge through coursework (C), verbal conversation (V), quizzes (Q), worksheets (W), or other approved activities (O).

2. Refine your knowledge through discussions with peer teachers and clinical instructors.

3. Demonstrate proficiency to a peer teacher and an ACI.

APPROVED BY
(date and signature, and mode for didactic)

1. Biochemistry/Physiology

    Didactic _____

    Peer _____

    ACI _____

2. Pharmocodynamics

    Didactic _____

    Peer _____

    ACI _____

3. Exercise effects

    Didactic _____

    Peer _____

    ACI _____

4. Administration modes

    Didactic _____

    Peer _____

    ACI _____

COMMENTS

_____

_____

_____

_____

_____

Medication Policies and Procedures

Objective

Demonstrate an understanding of the medication policies and procedures of your institution, including tracking medications dispensed to athletes.

NATA Athletic Training Educational Competencies embedded in this module: PH-C1, PH-C2, PH-C11, PH-P1, PH-P2

Competencies

1. Explain the main points of your state's laws governing prescriptions and dispensing prescription and over-the-counter (OTC) medications.

2. Obtain a copy of the medication section of your institution's athletic training policies and procedures manual. Discuss these policies, including the following:

   a. Established protocols for use of OTC medications
   b. The types of OTC medications to be used according to the physical ailment
   c. How to identify the precautions, expiration date, lot number, and dosage of medications as provided on the package and individual dose packets
   d. Verbal and written instructions given to patients when administering OTC medication
   e. Documentation required when administering OTC medication

3. Document the tracking of medications by recording the following information about the medication:

   a. Name of athlete
   b. Date medication given
   c. Name of medication
   d. Manufacturer
   e. Amount
   f. Dosage
   g. Lot number
   h. Expiration date

Proficiency Demonstration

1. Develop appropriate subject knowledge through coursework (C), verbal conversation (V), quizzes (Q), worksheets (W), or other approved activities (O).

2. Refine your knowledge through discussions with peer teachers and clinical instructors.

3. Demonstrate proficiency to a peer teacher and an ACI.

APPROVED BY
(date and signature, and mode for didactic)

1. Legal implications
   Didactic _____
   Peer _____
   ACI _____

2. Policies and procedures
   Didactic _____
   Peer _____
   ACI _____

3. Documentation
   Didactic _____
   Peer _____
   ACI _____

COMMENTS

_____

_____

_____

_____

Basic Performance Nutrition and Supplementation

Objective

Demonstrate knowledge of basic nutritional and supplementation guidelines for athletes.

NATA Athletic Training Educational Competencies embedded in this module: NU-C2, NU-C3, NU-C4, NU-C5, NU-C6, NU-C7, CU-C8, NU-C9, NU-C10, NU-C11, NU-C12, NU-C13, CU-C15, NU-C16, NU-C17, NU-C19, NU-C20, NU-P2, NU-P3, NU-CP1, PH-C10, PH-C11, PH-P1

Competencies

1. Discuss the following, including their role in health, intake values for male and female athletes, and medical and musculoskeletal consequences of improper amounts (less and more) of each. Also discuss the signs and symptoms of improper amounts.

a. Recommended daily allowance (RDA) or equivalency
b. Protein intake
c. Fat intake
d. Carbohydrate intake
e. Vitamin intake
f. Mineral intake
g. Fluid intake
h. Macronutrients
i. Micronutrients

2. Calculate the basal metabolic rate (BMR) of energy expenditure for the following:

a. Female gymnast
b. Football linebacker
c. Distance swimmer
d. Athlete rehabilitating from ACL reconstruction

3. Using standard resources, calculate the energy expenditure and optimal caloric intake of the athletes in competency 2.

4. Using the RDA and MyPyramid food guide, discuss nutritional guidelines and recommend an appropriate dietary regimen for each of the athletes in competency 2.

5. Discuss digestion, absorption, and assimilation of fluids, foods, and common nutritional supplements, including the typical time course of each and the effects of exercise and nonexercise stresses on the process and time course.

6. Discuss the effect of items in competency 5 on the content and scheduling of meals both before and after practice and competition.

7. Demonstrate the ability to access current nutritional guidelines and information from position papers by professional organizations, scientific research, and governmental agencies to address the following situations:

a. Nutritional supplements
b. Weight loss
c. Weight gain
d. Fluid replacement

8. Access appropriate informational resources that detail the advantages and disadvantages of nutritional supplements and performance-enhancing substances.

9. Obtain lists of banned substances (including nutritional supplements) for athletes at various levels of competition (e.g., high school, NCAA), and detail the consequences of improper use, abuse, or misuse by athletes at each level.

Proficiency Demonstration

1. Develop appropriate subject knowledge through coursework (C), verbal conversation (V), quizzes (Q), worksheets (W), or other approved activities (O).

2. Refine your knowledge through discussions with peer teachers and clinical instructors.

3. Demonstrate proficiency to a peer teacher and an ACI.

APPROVED BY
(date and signature, and mode for didactic)

1. Intake values

Didactic _____

Peer _____

ACI _____

2. BMR

Didactic _____

Peer _____

ACI _____

3. Energy expenditure and intake

Didactic _____

Peer _____

ACI _____

4. Nutritional guidelines and recommended regimen

Didactic _____

Peer _____

ACI _____

5. Digestion

Didactic _____

Peer _____

ACI _____

6. Pre- and postactivity meals

Didactic _____

Peer _____

ACI _____

7. Accessing nutritional guidelines and information

Didactic _____

Peer _____

ACI _____

8. Accessing resources for nutritional supplements and performance-enhancing substances

Didactic _____

Peer _____

ACI _____

9. Banned substances

Didactic _____

Peer _____

ACI _____

COMMENTS

_____

_____

_____

_____

Eating Disorders

Objective

Demonstrate a knowledge of eating disorders and the ability to intervene with athletes who suffer from such disorders.

NATA Athletic Training Educational Competencies embedded in this module: NU-C5, NU-C14, NU-CP2, ?-C10, MC-C18

Competencies

1. Define the following eating disorders and identify their common signs and symptoms:

   a. Anorexia
   b. Bulimia
   c. Obesity

2. Identify the physical and psychological consequences of the eating disorders in competency 1.

3. Simulate intervention with an athlete who has the signs and symptoms of disordered eating.

4. Identify proper referral sources for disordered eating.

Proficiency Demonstration

1. Develop appropriate subject knowledge through coursework (C), verbal conversation (V), quizzes (Q), worksheets (W), or other approved activities (O).

2. Refine your knowledge through discussions with peer teachers and clinical instructors.

3. Demonstrate proficiency to a peer teacher and an ACI.

APPROVED BY
(date and signature, and mode for didactic)

  a. Anorexia

   Didactic _____

   Peer _____

   ACI _____

1b. Bulimia

   Didactic _____

   Lab _____

   Peer _____

   ACI _____

1c. Obesity

   Didactic _____

   Peer _____

   ACI _____

2. Consequences

   Didactic _____

   Peer _____

   ACI _____

3. Intervention

   Didactic _____

   Peer _____

   ACI _____

4. Referral

   Didactic _____

   Peer _____

   ACI _____

COMMENTS

_____

_____

_____

_____

Health and Wellness

Objective

Develop and demonstrate understanding of current concepts of health and wellness as they apply to the daily practice of ATs and their interaction with physically active people.

NATA Athletic Training Educational Competencies embedded in this module: NU-C1, NU-C2, NU-C3, NU-C5, NU-C10, NU-C11, NU-C12, NU-P3, RM-C6

Competencies

1. Describe the general principles of the following:
   a. MyPyramid nutritional information
   b. The role of the FDA in regulation and control of nutritional and supplemental products
   c. The role of nutrition, exercise, and supplements in weight control

2. Discuss why and how a person maintains a healthy lifestyle through personal health habits such as the following:
   a. Personal hygiene
   b. Skin care
   c. Dental hygiene
   d. Sanitation
   e. Immunizations
   f. Injury and illness prevention
   g. Rest and sleep habits
   h. Exercise
   i. Weight control

3. Explain where to locate resources for nutritional information, including position papers of professional organizations, scientific research, and governmental agencies.

4. Describe the relationship between poor nutrition and orthopedic injuries, illnesses, diseases, and other health issues.

5. Develop pamphlets, handouts, presentations, posters, and so on that can be used to disseminate nutritional information to athletes and physically active people of all ages.

Proficiency Demonstration

1. Develop appropriate subject knowledge through coursework (C), verbal conversation (V), quizzes (Q), worksheets (W), or other approved activities (O).

2. Refine your knowledge through discussions with peer teachers and clinical instructors.

3. Demonstrate proficiency to a peer teacher and an ACI.

APPROVED BY
(date and signature, and mode for didactic)

1a. MyPyramid
   Didactic _____
   Peer _____
   ACI _____

1b. FDA roles
   Didactic _____
   Peer _____
   ACI _____

1c. Nutrition, exercise, and supplements
   Didactic _____
   Peer _____
   ACI _____

2a. Personal hygiene
   Didactic _____
   Peer _____
   ACI _____

2b. Skin care
   Didactic _____
   Peer _____
   ACI _____

2c. Dental hygiene
   Didactic _____
   Peer _____
   ACI _____

2d. Sanitation
   Didactic _____
   Peer _____
   ACI _____

2e. Immunizations
   Didactic _____
   Peer _____
   ACI _____

2f. Injury and illness prevention

Didactic _____

Peer _____

ACI _____

2g. Rest and sleep habits

Didactic _____

Peer _____

ACI _____

2h. Exercise

Didactic _____

Peer _____

ACI _____

2i. Weight control

Didactic _____

Peer _____

ACI _____

3. Locating resources

Didactic _____

Peer _____

ACI _____

4. Relationship between poor nutrition and health

Didactic _____

Peer _____

ACI _____

5. Developing educational material

Didactic _____

Peer _____

ACI _____

COMMENTS

_____

_____

_____

_____

_____

_____

General Assessment and Evaluation

We do not expect a car mechanic to respond to our complaints of a poorly running car by changing the oil, rotating the tires, or filling it up with gas in hopes that one of those responses might correct the problem. In some cases this random approach may work—sometimes even a blind squirrel finds a nut. Nonetheless, in most cases this random attempt at correcting the complaint will fall short. Proper and timely auto repair is facilitated when diagnostic and functional tests are performed to determine the exact cause of the problem, allowing the mechanic to begin the process of correcting it.

Similarly, athletic trainers are called upon to address patient complaints by first thoroughly assessing their physical status and then applying appropriate clinical interventions. Knowledge of assessment and testing procedures provides athletic trainers with information that can then be used in clinical decision making to facilitate recovery. By examining the skeletal system, laxity of ligaments, muscle strength, innervations, posture, ROM, strength, cardio-respiratory fitness, organ function, or general medical status, the athletic trainer obtains objective evidence that facilitates future care. Poor assessment techniques can lead to inappropriate care responses, wasted time, and poorly directed care.

In the following modules, students will begin to learn, practice, and implement general assessment techniques that will be used to varying degrees during evaluations of specific complaints, injuries, and illnesses. Knowledge of these general principles will serve as the foundation for more specific injury and illness assessments addressed in future modules.

Orthopedic Injury Assessment Principles

Objective

Demonstrate understanding of various techniques, diagnostic procedures, assessment tools, and tests used to evaluate common injuries caused by the risk factors associated with physical activity.

NATA Athletic Training Educational Competencies embedded in this module: DI-C6, DI-C7, DI-C9, DI-C10, DI-C11, DI-C12, DI-C13 DI-C15, DI-C17, DI-P10, MC-P1, MC-P2, MC-P3, MC-CP1

Competencies

1. Explain the differences among stress, special, and functional tests.

2. Describe the components of SOAP, HIPS, and HOPS injury assessment and documentation.

3. Discuss the purpose of and common procedures used to accomplish the following during injury assessment and diagnosis.

  a. History of person and of the current incident
  b. Observation and inspection of the entire body and specific abnormalities
  c. Preliminary diagnosis based on history and observation
  d. Palpation of suspected noninjured and injured body parts
  e. Range of motion via passive and active ROM
  f. Joint integrity via passive ROM and special tests
  g. Muscle function via resistive ROM, break tests, and manual muscle testing
  h. Circulatory status
  i. Neurological status of cranial, sensory, and motor nerves
  j. Posture and gait
  k. Diagnostic and imaging tests prescribed by a physician
  l. Documentation of results

4. Assess and diagnose an injured patient using the techniques and procedures in competency 3.

5. Explain the impact of psychological factors, such as malingering, pain tolerance, hypochondria, and so on, and their impact on injury assessment and evaluation.

6. Discuss risk factors inherent in various sporting activities so that you can determine appropriate functional testing.

7. Demonstrate understanding of the importance of ergonomic considerations during injury assessment.

Proficiency Demonstration

1. Develop appropriate subject knowledge through coursework (C), verbal conversation (V), quizzes (Q), worksheets (W), or other approved activities (O).

2. Practice and reinforce the skills in clinical skills and laboratory courses.

3. Refine your skills by observing peer teachers and clinical instructors as they perform the skills (preferably on patients), discussing the competencies with peer teachers and clinical instructors, practicing alone and with others, and then demonstrating proficiency to a peer teacher.

4. Demonstrate your proficiency to an ACI.

APPROVED BY
(date and signature, and mode for didactic)

1. Tests

   Didactic _____

   Lab _____

   Peer _____

   ACI _____

2. SOAP, HIPS, and HOPS

   Didactic _____

   Lab _____

   Peer _____

   ACI _____

3a. Purpose and techniques—history

   Didactic _____

   Lab _____

   Peer _____

   ACI _____

3b. Purpose and techniques—observation and inspection

   Didactic _____

   Lab _____

   Peer _____

   ACI _____

3c. Purpose and techniques—preliminary diagnosis

Didactic _____

Lab _____

Peer _____

ACI _____

3d. Purpose and techniques—palpation

Didactic _____

Lab _____

Peer _____

ACI _____

3e. Purpose and techniques—ROM

Didactic _____

Lab _____

Peer _____

ACI _____

3f. Purpose and techniques—joint integrity

Didactic _____

Lab _____

Peer _____

ACI _____

3g. Purpose and techniques—muscle function

Didactic _____

Lab _____

Peer _____

ACI _____

3h. Purpose and techniques—circulatory status

Didactic _____

Lab _____

Peer _____

ACI _____

3i. Purpose and techniques—neurological status

Didactic _____

Lab _____

Peer _____

ACI _____

3j. Purpose and techniques—posture and gait

Didactic _____

Lab _____

Peer _____

ACI _____

3k. Purpose and techniques—diagnostic and imaging tests

Didactic _____

Lab _____

Peer _____

ACI _____

3l. Purpose and techniques—documentation of results

Didactic _____

Lab _____

Peer _____

ACI _____

4. Injury assessment

Didactic _____

Lab _____

Peer _____

ACI _____

5. Psychological factors

Didactic _____

Lab _____

Peer _____

ACI _____

6. Risk factors

Didactic _____

Lab _____

Peer _____

ACI _____

7. Ergonomics

Didactic _____

Lab _____

Peer _____

ACI _____

COMMENTS

_____

_____

General Medical Assessment

Objective

Demonstrate the ability to assess a person's general medical status.

NATA Athletic Training Educational Competencies embedded in this module: MC-C3, MC-C22, MC-P1, MC-P2, MC-P3, MC-P4, MC-CP1, AC-C7, DI-P1

Competencies

1. Take a basic medical history that includes at least the following components:

  a. Previous medical history
  b. Previous surgical history
  c. Pertinent family medical history
  d. Current medication history
  e. Relevant social history
  f. Chief medical complaint

2. Measure body temperature via the following methods. Tell how they each relate to core temperature and to each other.

  a. Oral temperature
  b. Axillary temperature
  c. Tympanic temperature
  d. Rectal temperature

3. Measure the following vital signs:

  a. Blood pressure
  b. Pulse (rate and quality)
  c. Respiration (rate and quality)

4. Palpate the abdominal quadrants. Tell how you would know if the patient experienced pain or guarding and rigidity during your palpation. What medical conditions do these signs indicate?

5. Identify the following with a stethoscope:

  a. Normal breath sounds
  b. Normal heart sounds
  c. Normal bowel sounds

6. Identify pathological breathing patterns associated with the following respiratory conditions. Tell how these can be used to make a differential assessment of the following respiratory conditions:

  a. Apnea
  b. Tachypnea
  c. Hyperventilation
  d. Bradypnea
  e. Dyspnea
  f. Obstructed airway

7. Use an otoscope to examine the nose and the outer and middle ear.

8. Measure urine values with Chemstrips (dipsticks). What are normal values, and what do abnormal values indicate?

Proficiency Demonstration

1. Develop appropriate subject knowledge through coursework (C), verbal conversation (V), quizzes (Q), worksheets (W), or other approved activities (O).

2. Practice and reinforce the skills in clinical skills and laboratory courses.

3. Refine your skills by observing peer teachers and clinical instructors as they perform the skills (preferably on patients), discussing the competencies with peer teachers and clinical instructors, practicing alone and with others, and then demonstrating proficiency to a peer teacher.

4. Demonstrate your proficiency to an ACI.

APPROVED BY
(date and signature, and mode for didactic)

1. General history

  Didactic _____

  Lab _____

  Peer _____

  ACI _____

2. Temperature

  Didactic _____

  Lab _____

  Peer _____

  ACI _____

3. Vital signs

  Didactic _____

  Lab _____

  Peer _____

  ACI _____

4. Palpating the abdominal quadrants

Didactic _____

Lab _____

Peer _____

ACI _____

5. Stethoscope use

Didactic _____

Lab _____

Peer _____

ACI _____

6. Breathing patterns

Didactic _____

Lab _____

Peer _____

ACI _____

7. Otoscope use

Didactic _____

Lab _____

Peer _____

ACI _____

8. Urine values

Didactic _____

Lab _____

Peer _____

ACI _____

COMMENTS

_____

_____

_____

_____

_____

_____

_____

Postural Assessment

Objective

Develop and demonstrate the skills necessary to assess normal and abnormal posture.

NATA Athletic Training Educational Competencies embedded in this module: RM-C11, DI-C4, DI-C11, DI-C15, DI-P3

Competencies

1. Perform a postural assessment of the following:
   a. Cervical spine and head
   b. Shoulder
   c. Lumbothoracic region
   d. Hip and pelvis
   e. Knee
   f. Ankle, foot, and toes

2. Identify the following postural deviations and tell how they can predispose a person to injury.
   a. Kyphosis
   b. Lordosis
   c. Scoliosis
   d. Pelvic obliquity
   e. Tibial torsion
   f. Hip anteversion and retroversion
   g. Genu valgum, varum, and recurvatum
   h. Rearfoot valgus and varus
   i. Forefoot valgus and varus
   j. Pes cavus and planus
   k. Foot and toe posture

3. Identify the characteristics of the following body types. Name three athletes at your institution who would be classified in each category.
   a. Endomorph
   b. Ectomorph
   c. Mesomorph

Proficiency Demonstration

1. Develop appropriate subject knowledge through coursework (C), verbal conversation (V), quizzes (Q), worksheets (W), or other approved activities (O).

2. Practice and reinforce the skills in clinical skills and laboratory courses.

3. Refine your skills by observing peer teachers and clinical instructors as they perform the skills (preferably on patients), discussing the competencies with peer teachers and clinical instructors, practicing alone and with others, and then demonstrating proficiency to a peer teacher.

4. Demonstrate your proficiency to an ACI.

APPROVED BY
(date and signature, and mode for didactic)

1. Postural assessment
   Didactic _____
   Lab _____
   Peer _____
   ACI _____

2. Postural deviations
   Didactic _____
   Lab _____
   Peer _____
   ACI _____

3. Body types
   Didactic _____
   Lab _____
   Peer _____
   ACI _____

COMMENTS

_____

_____

_____

_____

_____

_____

_____

Neurological Assessment

Objective

Develop and demonstrate the skills necessary to identify and assess general neurological structure and function.

NATA Athletic Training Educational Competencies embedded in this module: DI-C8, DI-C9, DI-P9, AC-P4

Competencies

Identify and assess the following:

  a. Cranial nerves

  b. Dermatomes

  c. Myotomes

  d. Deep tendon reflexes

  e. Pathological reflexes

Proficiency Demonstration

1. Develop appropriate subject knowledge through coursework (C), verbal conversation (V), quizzes (Q), worksheets (W), or other approved activities (O).

2. Practice and reinforce the skills in clinical skills and laboratory courses.

3. Refine your skills by observing peer teachers and clinical instructors as they perform the skills (preferably on patients), discussing the competencies with peer teachers and clinical instructors, practicing alone and with others, and then demonstrating proficiency to a peer teacher.

4. Demonstrate your proficiency to an ACI.

APPROVED BY
(date and signature, and mode for didactic)

  1a. Cranial nerves

    Didactic _____

    Lab _____

    Peer _____

    ACI _____

  1b. Dermatomes

    Didactic _____

    Lab _____

    Peer _____

    ACI _____

  1c. Myotomes

    Didactic _____

    Lab _____

    Peer _____

    ACI _____

  1d. Deep tendon reflexes

    Didactic _____

    Lab _____

    Peer _____

    ACI _____

  1e. Pathological reflexes

    Didactic _____

    Lab _____

    Peer _____

    ACI _____

COMMENTS

_____

_____

_____

_____

_____

_____

_____

_____

_____

Palpation

Objective

Develop and demonstrate the skills necessary to palpate anatomical structures.

NATA Athletic Training Educational Competencies embedded in this module: DI-C6, DI-P4, MC-P3

Competencies

Identify the following by palpation:

a. Bony landmarks of the head, trunk, spine, scapula, and extremities

b. Soft tissue structures of the head, trunk, spine, and extremities

c. Abdominal and thoracic structures

d. Primary neurological and circulatory structures

Proficiency Demonstration

1. Develop appropriate subject knowledge through coursework (C), verbal conversation (V), quizzes (Q), worksheets (W), or other approved activities (O).

2. Practice and reinforce the skills in clinical skills and laboratory courses.

3. Refine your skills by observing peer teachers and clinical instructors as they perform the skills (preferably on patients), discussing the competencies with peer teachers and clinical instructors, practicing alone and with others, and then demonstrating proficiency to a peer teacher.

4. Demonstrate your proficiency to an ACI.

APPROVED BY
(date and signature, and mode for didactic)

1a. Bony landmarks

Didactic _____

Lab _____

Peer _____

ACI _____

1b. Soft tissue structures

Didactic _____

Lab _____

Peer _____

ACI _____

1c. Abdominal and thoracic structures

Didactic _____

Lab _____

Peer _____

ACI _____

1d. Neurological and circulatory structures

Didactic _____

Lab _____

Peer _____

ACI _____

COMMENTS

_____

_____

_____

_____

_____

_____

Range-of-Motion and Strength Assessment

Objective

Develop and demonstrate the skills necessary to assess ROM and manual muscle strength.

NATA Athletic Training Educational Competencies embedded in this module: DI-C12, DI-P5, DI-P6, EX-C7, EX-P2

Competencies

1. Using both a goniometer and an inclinometer, quantitatively assess active and passive ROM of the following:

    a. Temporomandibular joint (TMJ)
    b. Cervical spine
    c. Shoulder
    d. Elbow
    e. Wrist and hand
    f. Thumb and fingers
    g. Hip
    h. Lumbar spine
    i. Thoracic spine
    j. Knee
    k. Ankle
    l. Foot and toes

2. Using manual muscle testing and break tests, qualitatively assess muscle strength of the structures in competency 1.

Proficiency Demonstration

1. Develop appropriate subject knowledge through coursework (C), verbal conversation (V), quizzes (Q), worksheets (W), or other approved activities (O).

2. Practice and reinforce the skills in clinical skills and laboratory courses.

3. Refine your skills by observing peer teachers and clinical instructors as they perform the skills (preferably on patients), discussing the competencies with peer teachers and clinical instructors, practicing alone and with others, and then demonstrating proficiency to a peer teacher.

4. Demonstrate your proficiency to an ACI.

APPROVED BY
(date and signature, and mode for didactic)

1a and 2a. TMJ

    Didactic _____

    Lab _____

    Peer _____

    ACI _____

1b and 2b. Cervical spine

    Didactic _____

    Lab _____

    Peer _____

    ACI _____

1c and 2c. Shoulder

    Didactic _____

    Lab _____

    Peer _____

    ACI _____

1d and 2d. Elbow

    Didactic _____

    Lab _____

    Peer _____

    ACI _____

1e and 2e. Wrist and hand

    Didactic _____

    Lab _____

    Peer _____

    ACI _____

1f and 2f. Thumb and fingers

    Didactic _____

    Lab _____

    Peer _____

    ACI _____

1g and 2g. Hip

    Didactic _____

    Lab _____

    Peer _____

    ACI _____

1h and 2h. Lumbar spine

    Didactic _____

    Lab _____

    Peer _____

    ACI _____

1i and 2i. Thoracic spine

    Didactic _____

    Lab _____

    Peer _____

    ACI _____

1j and 2j. Knee

    Didactic _____

    Lab _____

    Peer _____

    ACI _____

1k and 2k. Ankle

    Didactic _____

    Lab _____

    Peer _____

    ACI _____

1l and 2l. Foot and toes

    Didactic _____

    Lab _____

    Peer _____

    ACI _____

COMMENTS

_____

_____

_____

_____

_____

Physical Performance Measurements

Objective

Develop and demonstrate the skills necessary to measure selected elements of physical performance.

NATA Athletic Training Educational Competencies embedded in this module: DI-C12, EX-C7, RM-C11, RM-C13, RM-P1

Competencies

1. Perform and interpret repetition maximum tests to measure the strength of the following:

    a. Elbow flexors
    b. Leg (leg press or squat)

2. Perform and interpret isokinetic tests to measure the strength of the following:

    a. Knee (extensors)
    b. Shoulder (press)

3. Perform and interpret isometric tests for the following:

    a. Ankle
    b. Foot and toes
    c. Knee
    d. Hip
    e. Torso
    f. Shoulder
    g. Elbow
    h. Wrist
    i. Hand and fingers

4. Perform and interpret the following tests:

    a. Upper-body strength test
    b. Lower-body strength test
    c. Upper-body power test
    d. Lower-body power test
    e. Upper-body muscular endurance test
    f. Lower-body muscular endurance test
    g. Agility
    h. Speed

Proficiency Demonstration

1. Develop appropriate subject knowledge through coursework (C), verbal conversation (V), quizzes (Q), worksheets (W), or other approved activities (O).

2. Practice and reinforce the skills in clinical skills and laboratory courses.

3. Refine your skills by observing peer teachers and clinical instructors as they perform the skills (preferably on patients), discussing the competencies with peer teachers and clinical instructors, practicing alone and with others, and then demonstrating proficiency to a peer teacher.

4. Demonstrate your proficiency to an ACI.

APPROVED BY
(date and signature, and mode for didactic)

1. Repetition maximum tests

    Didactic _____

    Lab _____

    Peer _____

    ACI _____

2. Isokinetic tests

    Didactic _____

    Lab _____

    Peer _____

    ACI _____

3. Isometric tests

    Didactic _____

    Lab _____

    Peer _____

    ACI _____

4a. Strength—upper body

    Didactic _____

    Lab _____

    Peer _____

    ACI _____

4b. Strength—lower body

    Didactic _____

    Lab _____

    Peer _____

    ACI _____

4c. Power—upper body

    Didactic _____

    Lab _____

    Peer _____

    ACI _____

4d. Power—lower body

Didactic _____

Lab _____

Peer _____

ACI _____

4e. Muscular endurance—upper body

Didactic _____

Lab _____

Peer _____

ACI _____

4f. Muscular endurance—lower body

Didactic _____

Lab _____

Peer _____

ACI _____

4g. Agility

Didactic _____

Lab _____

Peer _____

ACI _____

4h. Speed

Didactic _____

Lab _____

Peer _____

ACI _____

COMMENTS

_____

_____

_____

_____

_____

_____

_____

Orthopedic Injury Assessment

Objective

Use various techniques, diagnostic procedures, assessment tools, and special tests to assess a common musculoskeletal injury.

NATA Athletic Training Educational Competencies embedded in this module: DI-P1, DI-P2, DI-P3, DI-P4, DI-P5, DI-P6, DI-P7, DI-P8, DI-P9, DI-P10

Competencies

After you have completed modules I1 through I7, use the following techniques to assess and diagnose a peer for an injury suggested by your lab instructor, and then assess and diagnose an injured patient.

- a. History of the person and of the current incident
- b. Observation and inspection of the entire body and specific abnormalities
- c. Preliminary diagnosis based on history and observation
- d. Palpation of suspected noninjured and injured body parts
- e. ROM via passive and active ROM
- f. Joint integrity via passive ROM and special tests
- g. Muscle function via resistive ROM, break tests, and manual muscle testing
- h. Circulatory status
- i. Neurological status of cranial, sensory, and motor nerves
- j. Posture and gait
- k. Diagnostic and imaging tests prescribed by a physician
- l. Documentation of results

Proficiency Demonstration

Perform the evaluation in a lab or clinical skills class and then on a patient.

APPROVED BY
(injury, date, and signature)

Orthopedic injury assessment

Lab _____

Peer _____

ACI _____

COMMENTS

_____

_____

_____

_____

_____

_____

_____

_____

Level 2.9

Specific Injury Assessment and Diagnosis

Much of what ATs do is based on accurate and timely diagnosis. Assessment of injuries and illnesses is a critical step in the rehabilitation process. A proper diagnosis based on information gathered during the previously reviewed general assessment procedures along with objective information from body-part-specific assessment procedures outlined in the following modules will focus the care, treatment, and exercise believed to be helpful in restoring a patient to preinjury status. The faster a diagnosis is obtained through proper injury assessment, the earlier rehabilitation can begin. Without the information gained from an adequate assessment, clinical interventions could be similar to throwing darts in the dark, which often miss their intended goal.

Several of the general assessment procedures are the same regardless of injury, illness, or complaint. However, in many cases, additional information needs to be assembled from specific evaluation procedures to obtain an accurate diagnosis. The skills needed to evaluate specific body parts are the focus of the following modules.

Foot Injury Assessment and Diagnosis

Objective

Develop and demonstrate the skills necessary to evaluate foot injuries.

NATA Athletic Training Educational Competencies embedded in this module: AC-C6, DI-C6, DI-C7, DI-C10, DI-C12, DI-C13, DI-C15, DI-C16, DI-C17, DI-P1, DI-P2, DI-P4, DI-P5, DI-P6, DI-P7, DI-P8, DI-P10, DI-CP1.

Anatomy and Conditions for This Module

A. Bones and Prominent Bony Features

- Calcaneus
- Talus
- Cuboid
- Navicular
- Cuneiforms
- Metatarsals
  - Styloid process of fifth metatarsal
  - Phalanges
  - Sesamoids

B. Articulations

- Subtalar
- Transverse tarsal
- Metatarsal phalangeal (MP)
- Distal *interphalangeal* (DIP) and proximal *interphalangeal* (PIP)

C. Ligaments

- Long plantar
- Lateral retinaculum

D. Muscles

- Anterior tibialis
- Flexor hallucis longus
- Flexor digitorum longus
- Posterior tibialis
- Extensor hallucis longus
- Extensor digitorum longus
- Peroneus longus
- Peroneus brevis
- Peroneus tertius
- Gastrocnemius
- Soleus

E. Other Structures

- Peroneal nerve (entire course)
- Tibial nerve (entire course)
- Pedal pulse

F. Special Tests

- Compression test
- Tap or percussion test
- Tinel's sign
- Interdigital neuroma (pencil) test
- Midtarsal (tarsal twist) test
- Long bone compression (toe-tap) test
- Feiss line (navicular drop) test
- Gait analysis

G. Injuries and Conditions

- Ingrown toenail (paronychia)
- Bunions
- Calluses and corns
- Blisters
- Neuroma
- Plantarflexed first ray
- Hammer toes
- Claw toes
- Sprained hallux
- Sprained digit
- Exostosis
- Tarsal tunnel syndrome
- Apophysitis (Sever's disease)
- Dislocation or subluxation
- Forefoot varus and valgus
- Equinus deformity
- Pes cavus and planus
- Rearfoot (hindfoot) varus and valgus
- Hallux rigidus
- Hallux valgus
- Morton's foot syndrome
- Arch strains
- Plantar fasciitis
- Heel bruise
- Bursitis
- Tendinitis

- Tenosynovitis
- Fracture
- Stress fracture
- Avulsion fracture
- Sinus tarsi syndrome

Competencies

Note: All procedures must be performed.

Anatomical Review and Assessment of Structural Integrity

1. Name and palpate each bone and bony structure in list A. Tell what differences you would expect to feel if the bone were fractured.

2. Palpate or draw the joint line for each articulation in list B. Then perform active and passive joint ROM tests using both qualitative and quantitative techniques (e.g., tape measure, goniometer, and inclinometer). Record the results of these tests using accepted forms and procedures.

3. Using surface anatomy, palpate or draw the origins and course of each ligament in list C.

4. Using surface anatomy, palpate the origin, insertion, and course of each muscle in list D. Also, tell the major function of each muscle.

5. Using surface anatomy, palpate each structure in list E.

Injury Assessment

6. Obtain the medical history of an athlete with a suspected foot injury.

7. Demonstrate proper administration and interpretation of the special tests in list F.

8. Demonstrate how you would observe and identify the clinical signs and symptoms associated with the injuries and conditions in list G.

9. Explain and demonstrate the mechanisms by which each injury in list G occurs. Name the three sports in which each injury is most likely to occur and explain any differences among the injury occurrences and mechanisms in those sports.

10. Demonstrate appropriate sensory, circulatory, and neurological tests for the injuries in list G.

11. Palpate and assess the integrity of the bones and soft tissues associated with each injury in list G.

12. Perform special tests to assess the integrity of the joints involved in each injury in list G and explain how you would interpret these tests.

13. Demonstrate the use of manual muscle testing and other tests as appropriate to assess the flexibility and strength of the muscles associated with each injury in list G.

14. Demonstrate functional and activity-specific tests to determine the integrity of each structure involved in each injury in list G.

Proficiency Demonstration

1. Develop appropriate subject knowledge through coursework (C), verbal conversation (V), quizzes (Q), worksheets (W), or other approved activities (O).

2. Practice and reinforce the skills in clinical skills and laboratory courses.

3. Refine your skills by observing peer teachers and clinical instructors as they perform the skills (preferably on patients), discussing the competencies with peer teachers and clinical instructors, practicing alone and with others, and then demonstrating proficiency to a peer teacher.

4. Demonstrate your proficiency to an ACI.

APPROVED BY
(date and signature, and mode for didactic)

1. Bones

Didactic _____

Lab _____

Peer _____

ACI _____

2. Articulations

Didactic _____

Lab _____

Peer _____

ACI _____

3. Ligaments

Didactic _____

Lab _____

Peer _____

ACI _____

4. Muscles

Didactic _____

Lab _____

Peer _____

ACI _____

5. Other structures

Didactic _____

Lab _____

Peer _____

ACI _____

6. History

Didactic _____

Lab _____

Peer _____

ACI _____

7. Special tests

Compression test

Didactic _____

Lab _____

Peer _____

ACI _____

Tap or percussion test

Didactic _____

Lab _____

Peer _____

ACI _____

Tinel's sign

Didactic _____

Lab _____

Peer _____

ACI _____

Interdigital neuroma (pencil) test

Didactic _____

Lab _____

Peer _____

ACI _____

Midtarsal (tarsal twist) test

Didactic _____

Lab _____

Peer _____

ACI _____

Long bone compression (toe-tap) test

Didactic _____

Lab _____

Peer _____

ACI _____

Feiss line (navicular drop) test

Didactic _____

Lab _____

Peer _____

ACI _____

Gait analysis

Didactic _____

Lab _____

Peer _____

ACI _____

8-18. Complete competencies 8 through 14 for the injuries or conditions in list G:

Ingrown toenail

Didactic _____

Lab _____

Peer _____

ACI _____

Bunions

Didactic _____

Lab _____

Peer _____

ACI _____

Calluses and corns

Didactic _____

Lab _____

Peer _____

ACI _____

Blisters

Didactic _____

Lab _____

Peer _____

ACI _____

Neuroma

Didactic _____

Lab _____

Peer _____

ACI _____

Plantarflexed first ray

Didactic _____

Lab _____

Peer _____

ACI _____

Hammer toes

Didactic _____

Lab _____

Peer _____

ACI _____

Claw toes

Didactic _____

Lab _____

Peer _____

ACI _____

Sprained hallux

Didactic _____

Lab _____

Peer _____

ACI _____

Sprained digit

Didactic _____

Lab _____

Peer _____

ACI _____

Exostosis

Didactic _____

Lab _____

Peer _____

ACI _____

Tarsal tunnel syndrome

Didactic _____

Lab _____

Peer _____

ACI _____

Apophysitis

Didactic _____

Lab _____

Peer _____

ACI _____

Dislocation or subluxation

Didactic _____

Lab _____

Peer _____

ACI _____

Forefoot varus and valgus

Didactic _____

Lab _____

Peer _____

ACI _____

Equinus deformity

Didactic _____

Lab _____

Peer _____

ACI _____

Pes cavus and planus

Didactic _____

Lab _____

Peer _____

ACI _____

Rearfoot (hindfoot) varus and valgus

Didactic _____

Lab _____

Peer _____

ACI _____

Hallux rigidus

Didactic _____

Lab _____

Peer _____

ACI _____

Hallux valgus

Didactic _____

Lab _____

Peer _____

ACI _____

Morton's foot syndrome

Didactic _____

Lab _____

Peer _____

ACI _____

Arch strains

Didactic _____

Lab _____

Peer _____

ACI _____

Plantar fasciitis

Didactic _____

Lab _____

Peer _____

ACI _____

Heel bruise

Didactic _____

Lab _____

Peer _____

ACI _____

Bursitis

Didactic _____

Lab _____

Peer _____

ACI _____

Tendinitis

Didactic _____

Lab _____

Peer _____

ACI _____

Tenosynovitis

Didactic _____

Lab _____

Peer _____

ACI _____

Fracture

Didactic _____

Lab _____

Peer _____

ACI _____

Stress fracture

Didactic _____

Lab _____

Peer _____

ACI _____

Avulsion fracture

Didactic _____

Lab _____

Peer _____

ACI _____

Sinus tarsi syndrome

Didactic _____

Lab _____

Peer _____

ACI _____

COMMENTS

_____

_____

_____

Ankle Injury Assessment and Diagnosis

Objective

Develop and demonstrate the skills necessary to evaluate ankle injuries.

NATA Athletic Training Educational Competencies embedded in this module: AC-C6, DI-C6, DI-C7, DI-C10, DI-C12, DI-C13, DI-C15, DI-C16, DI-C17, DI-P1, DI-P2, DI-P4, DI-P5, DI-P6, DI-P7, DI-P8, DI-P10, DI-CP1

Anatomy and Conditions for This Module

A. Bones and Prominent Bony Features

- Calcaneus
- Talus
- Cuboid
- Navicular
- Cuneiforms
- Tibia
- Fibula

B. Articulations

- Ankle mortice
- Distal tibiofibular
- Subtalar
- Transverse tarsal

C. Ligaments

- Anterior talofibular
- Calcaneofibular
- Posterior talofibular
- Distal anterior tibiofibular
- Distal posterior tibiofibular
- Deltoid
- Peroneal retinaculum

D. Muscles

- Anterior tibialis
- Flexor hallucis longus
- Flexor digitorum longus
- Posterior tibialis
- Extensor hallucis longus
- Extensor digitorum longus
- Peroneus longus
- Peroneus brevis
- Peroneus tertius
- Gastrocnemius
- Soleus

E. Other Structures

- Anterior tibial artery
- Deep peroneal nerve
- Superficial peroneal nerve
- Posterior tibial

F. Special Tests

- Anterior drawer test
- Talar tilt test (inversion and eversion)
- Kleiger's (external rotation) test
- Tap or percussion test

G. Injuries and Conditions

- First-degree ankle sprain
- Second-degree ankle sprain
- Third-degree ankle sprain
- Sprain and dislocation
- Anterior tibialis strain
- Peroneal strain
- Fracture
- Stress fracture
- Avulsion fracture

Competencies

Note: All procedures must be performed.

Anatomical Review and Assessment of Structural Integrity

1. Name and palpate each bone and bony structure in list A. Tell what differences you would expect to feel if the bone were fractured.

2. Palpate or draw the joint line for each articulation in list B. Then perform active and passive joint ROM tests using both qualitative and quantitative techniques (e.g., tape measure, goniometer, and inclinometer). Record the results of these tests using accepted forms and procedures.

3. Using surface anatomy, palpate or draw the origins and course of each ligament in list C.

4. Using surface anatomy, palpate the origin, insertion, and course of each muscle in list D. Also, tell the major function of each muscle.

5. Using surface anatomy, palpate each structure in list E.

Injury Assessment

6. Obtain the medical history of an athlete with a suspected ankle injury.

7. Demonstrate proper administration and interpretation of the special tests in list F.

8. Demonstrate how you would observe and identify the clinical signs and symptoms associated with the injuries and conditions in list G.

9. Explain and demonstrate the mechanisms by which each injury in list G occurs. Name the three sports in which each injury is most likely to occur and explain any differences among the injury occurrences and mechanisms in those sports.

10. Demonstrate appropriate sensory, circulatory, and neurological tests for the injuries in list G.

11. Palpate and assess the integrity of the bones and soft tissues associated with each injury in list G.

12. Perform special tests to assess the integrity of the joints involved in each injury in list G and explain how you would interpret these tests.

13. Demonstrate the use of manual muscle testing and other tests as appropriate to assess the flexibility and strength of the muscles associated with each injury in list G.

14. Demonstrate functional and activity-specific tests to determine the integrity of each structure involved in each injury in list G.

Proficiency Demonstration

1. Develop appropriate subject knowledge through coursework (C), verbal conversation (V), quizzes (Q), worksheets (W), or other approved activities (O).

2. Practice and reinforce the skills in clinical skills and laboratory courses.

3. Refine your skills by observing peer teachers and clinical instructors as they perform the skills (preferably on patients), discussing the competencies with peer teachers and clinical instructors, practicing alone and with others, and then demonstrating proficiency to a peer teacher.

4. Demonstrate your proficiency to an ACI.

APPROVED BY
(date and signature, and mode for didactic)

1. Bones

   Didactic _____

   Lab _____

   Peer _____

   ACI _____

2. Articulations

   Didactic _____

   Lab _____

   Peer _____

   ACI _____

3. Ligaments

   Didactic _____

   Lab _____

   Peer _____

   ACI _____

4. Muscles

   Didactic _____

   Lab _____

   Peer _____

   ACI _____

5. Other structures

   Didactic _____

   Lab _____

   Peer _____

   ACI _____

6. History

   Didactic _____

   Lab _____

   Peer _____

   ACI _____

7. Special tests

   Anterior drawer test

   Didactic _____

   Lab _____

   Peer _____

   ACI _____

Talar tilt test (inversion and eversion)

Didactic _____

Lab _____

Peer _____

ACI _____

Kleiger's (external rotation) test

Didactic _____

Lab _____

Peer _____

ACI _____

Tap or percussion test

Didactic _____

Lab _____

Peer _____

ACI _____

8-14. Complete competencies 8 through 14 for the injuries or conditions in list G:

First-degree ankle sprain

Didactic _____

Lab _____

Peer _____

ACI _____

Second-degree ankle sprain

Didactic _____

Lab _____

Peer _____

ACI _____

Third-degree ankle sprain

Didactic _____

Lab _____

Peer _____

ACI _____

Sprain and dislocation

Didactic _____

Lab _____

Peer _____

ACI _____

Anterior tibialis strain

Didactic _____

Lab _____

Peer _____

ACI _____

Peroneal strain

Didactic _____

Lab _____

Peer _____

ACI _____

Fracture

Didactic _____

Lab _____

Peer _____

ACI _____

Stress fracture

Didactic _____

Lab _____

Peer _____

ACI _____

Avulsion fracture

Didactic _____

Lab _____

Peer _____

ACI _____

COMMENTS

_____

_____

_____

_____

_____

Lower-Leg Injury Assessment and Diagnosis

Objective

Develop and demonstrate the skills necessary to evaluate lower-leg injuries.

NATA Athletic Training Educational Competencies embedded in this module: DI-C6, DI-C7, DI-C10, DI-C12, DI-C13, DI-C15, DI-C16, DI-C17, DI-P1, DI-P2, DI-P4, DI-P5, DI-P6, DI-P7, DI-P8, DI-P10, DI-CP1, AC-C6

Anatomy and Conditions for This Module

A. Bones and Prominent Bony Features

- Tibia
  - Anterior border
  - Medial condyle
  - Lateral condyle
  - Gerdy's tubercle
  - Patellar tubercle
  - Malleolus
- Fibula
  - Head
  - Shaft
  - Malleolus

B. Articulations

- Proximal tibiofibular
- Distal tibiofibular

C. Ligaments

- Interosseous ligament
- Anterior tibio-fibular ligament
- Posterior tibio-fibular ligament

D. Muscles

- Anterior tibialis
- Posterior tibialis
- Flexor hallucis longus
- Flexor digitorum longus
- Extensor hallucis longus
- Extensor digitorum longus
- Peroneus longus
- Peroneus tertius
- Gastrocnemius
- Soleus

E. Other Structures

- Common peroneal nerve (entire course)
- Pedal pulse

F. Special Tests

- Homans' sign
- Thompson's test
- Tap or percussion test
- Tibiofibular translation test

G. Injuries and Conditions

- Achilles tendon strain or rupture
- Achilles bursitis and tenosynovitis
- Anterior shin splints
- Posterior shin splints
- Compartment syndrome
- Muscular strain and rupture
- Contusion
- Peroneal nerve contusion
- Fracture
- Stress fracture
- Tibial stress syndrome
- Fasciitis
- Osteochondritis dissecans
- Deep vein thrombosis

Competencies

Note: All procedures must be performed.

Anatomical Review and Assessment of Structural Integrity

1. Name and palpate each bone and bony structure in list A. Tell what differences you would expect to feel if the bone were fractured.

2. Palpate or draw the joint line for each articulation in list B. Then perform active and passive joint ROM tests using both qualitative and quantitative techniques (e.g., tape measure, goniometer, and inclinometer). Record the results of these tests using accepted forms and procedures.

3. Using surface anatomy, palpate or draw the origins and course of each ligament in list C.

4. Using surface anatomy, palpate the origin, insertion, and course of each muscle in list D. Also, tell the major function of each muscle.

5. Using surface anatomy, palpate each structure in list E.

Injury Assessment

6. Obtain the medical history of an athlete with a suspected lower-leg injury.

7. Demonstrate proper administration and interpretation of the special tests in list F.

8. Demonstrate how you would observe and identify the clinical signs and symptoms associated with the injuries and conditions in list G.

9. Explain and demonstrate the mechanisms by which each injury in list G occurs. Name the three sports in which each injury is most likely to occur and explain any differences among the injury occurrences and mechanisms in those sports.

10. Demonstrate appropriate sensory, circulatory, and neurological tests for the injuries in list G.

11. Palpate and assess the integrity of the bones and soft tissues associated with each injury in list G.

12. Perform special tests to assess the integrity of the joints involved in each injury in list G and explain how you would interpret these tests.

13. Demonstrate the use of manual muscle testing and other tests as appropriate to assess the flexibility and strength of the muscles associated with each injury in list G.

14. Demonstrate functional and activity-specific tests to determine the integrity of each structure involved in each injury in list G.

Proficiency Demonstration

1. Develop appropriate subject knowledge through coursework (C), verbal conversation (V), quizzes (Q), worksheets (W), or other approved activities (O).

2. Practice and reinforce the skills in clinical skills and laboratory courses.

3. Refine your skills by observing peer teachers and clinical instructors as they perform the skills (preferably on patients), discussing the competencies with peer teachers and clinical instructors, practicing alone and with others, and then demonstrating proficiency to a peer teacher.

4. Demonstrate your proficiency to an ACI.

APPROVED BY
(date and signature, and mode for didactic)

1. Bones
Didactic _____
Lab _____
Peer _____
ACI _____

2. Articulations
Didactic _____
Lab _____
Peer _____
ACI _____

3. Ligaments
Didactic _____
Lab _____
Peer _____
ACI _____

4. Muscles
Didactic _____
Lab _____
Peer _____
ACI _____

5. Other structures
Didactic _____
Lab _____
Peer _____
ACI _____

6. History
Didactic _____
Lab _____
Peer _____
ACI _____

7. Special tests
Homans' sign
Didactic _____
Lab _____
Peer _____
ACI _____

LEVEL
2.9

MODULE
J3

Thompson's test

Didactic _____

Lab _____

Peer _____

ACI _____

Tap or percussion test

Didactic _____

Lab _____

Peer _____

ACI _____

Tibiofibular translation test

Didactic _____

Lab _____

Peer _____

ACI _____

8-14. Complete competencies 8 through 14 for the injuries or conditions in list G:

Achilles strain or rupture

Didactic _____

Lab _____

Peer _____

ACI _____

Achilles bursitis and tenosynovitis

Didactic _____

Lab _____

Peer _____

ACI _____

Anterior shin splints

Didactic _____

Lab _____

Peer _____

ACI _____

Posterior shin splints

Didactic _____

Lab _____

Peer _____

ACI _____

Compartment syndrome

Didactic _____

Lab _____

Peer _____

ACI _____

Muscular strain and rupture

Didactic _____

Lab _____

Peer _____

ACI _____

Contusion

Didactic _____

Lab _____

Peer _____

ACI _____

Peroneal nerve contusion

Didactic _____

Lab _____

Peer _____

ACI _____

Fracture

Didactic _____

Lab _____

Peer _____

ACI _____

Stress fracture

Didactic _____

Lab _____

Peer _____

ACI _____

Tibial stress syndrome

Didactic _____

Lab _____

Peer _____

ACI _____

Fasciitis

Didactic _____

Lab _____

Peer _____

ACI _____

Osteochondritis dissecans

Didactic _____

Lab _____

Peer _____

ACI _____

Deep vein thrombosis

Didactic _____

Lab _____

Peer _____

ACI _____

COMMENTS

_____

_____

_____

_____

_____

_____

_____

Knee Injury Assessment and Diagnosis

Objective

Develop and demonstrate the skills necessary to evaluate knee injuries.

NATA Athletic Training Educational Competencies embedded in this module: AC-C6, DI-C6, DI-C7, DI-C10, DI-C12, DI-C13, DI-C15, DI-C16, DI-C17, DI-P1, DI-P2, DI-P4, DI-P5, DI-P6, DI-P7, DI-P8, DI-P10, DI-CP1

Anatomy and Conditions for This Module

A. Bones and Prominent Bony Features

- Femur
  - Condyles
  - Epicondyles
- Tibia
  - Medial condyle
  - Lateral condyle
  - Gerdy's tubercle
- Fibula
  - Head
  - Proximal shaft
- Patella

B. Articulations

- Medial tibiofemoral
- Lateral tibiofemoral
- Superior tibiofibular
- Tibiofemoral

C. Ligaments

- Lateral capsular
- Lateral collateral
- Medial capsular (deep collateral)
- Posterior fibers
- Middle fibers
- Anterior fibers
- Medial collateral (superficial collateral)
- Anterior cruciate
- Posterior cruciate
- Quadriceps tendon
- Patellar

D. Muscles

- Biceps femoris (long and short heads)
- Semitendinosus
- Semimembranosus
- Rectus femoris
- Vastus medialis
- Vastus intermedius
- Vastus lateralis
- Sartorius
- Tensor fasciae latae
- Iliotibial band
- Gracilis
- Gastrocnemius (medial and lateral heads)
- Popliteus

E. Other Structures

- Common peroneal nerve
- Popliteal artery
- Suprapatellar bursa
- Patellar bursa
- Infrapatellar fat pad
- Infrapatellar bursa
- Superficial bursa

F. Special Tests

- Observation of tibiofemoral and patellar alignment
- Patellar glide, tilt, and rotation test
- Valgus stress test
- Varus stress test
- Lachman's test
- Anterior drawer test
- Posterior drawer test
- Slocum test
- Bounce home test
- Godfrey 90/90 test
- Posterior sag (profile) sign
- Hughston's test
- Lateral pivot shift
- McMurray test
- Apley's compression and distraction test
- Thessaly test
- Patellar apprehension test
- Sweep test
- Ballottable patella

G. Injuries and Conditions

- Torn medial meniscus
- Torn lateral meniscus
- ACL sprain
- PCL sprain
- MCL sprain (superficial)
- MCL sprain (deep)
- LCL sprain
- Anteromedial rotary instability (AMRI)
- Anterolateral rotary instability (ALRI)
- Bursitis
- Capsular sprain
- Contused vastus medialis
- Patellofemoral joint pain
- Patellar tendinitis
- Patellar tendinosis
- Patellar tenosynovitis
- Fractured patella
- Baker's cyst
- Synovial plica
- Hyperextended knee
- Osgood-Schlatter disease
- Iliotibial band syndrome
- Distal hamstring strain
- Chondromalacia patella
- Patellar dislocation and subluxation
- Fat pad contusion
- Fracture
- Osteochondritis dissecans
- Patellar tendon rupture
- Peroneal nerve contusion or palsy
- Tendinitis
- Tibial torsion

Competencies

Note: All procedures must be performed.

Anatomical Review and Assessment of Structural Integrity

1. Name and palpate each bone and bony structure in list A. Tell what differences you would expect to feel if the bone were fractured.

2. Palpate or draw the joint line for each articulation in list B. Then perform active and passive joint ROM tests using both qualitative and quantitative techniques (e.g., tape measure, goniometer, and inclinometer). Record the results of these tests using accepted forms and procedures.

3. Using surface anatomy, palpate or draw the origins and course of each ligament in list C.

4. Using surface anatomy, palpate the origin, insertion, and course of each muscle in list D. Also, tell the major function of each muscle.

5. Using surface anatomy, palpate each structure in list E.

Injury Assessment

6. Obtain the medical history of an athlete with a suspected knee injury.

7. Demonstrate proper administration and interpretation of the special tests in list F.

8. Demonstrate how you would observe and identify the clinical signs and symptoms associated with the injuries and conditions in list G.

9. Explain and demonstrate the mechanisms by which each injury in list G occurs. Name the three sports in which each injury is most likely to occur and explain any differences among the injury occurrences and mechanisms in those sports.

10. Demonstrate appropriate sensory, circulatory, and neurological tests for the injuries in list G.

11. Palpate and assess the integrity of the bones and soft tissues associated with each injury in list G.

12. Perform special tests to assess the integrity of the joints involved in each injury in list G and explain how you would interpret these tests.

13. Demonstrate the use of manual muscle testing and other tests as appropriate to assess the flexibility and strength of the muscles associated with each injury in list G.

14. Demonstrate functional and activity-specific tests to determine the integrity of each structure involved in each injury in list G.

Proficiency Demonstration

1. Develop appropriate subject knowledge through coursework (C), verbal conversation (V), quizzes (Q), worksheets (W), or other approved activities (O).

2. Practice and reinforce the skills in clinical skills and laboratory courses.

3. Refine your skills by observing peer teachers and clinical instructors as they perform the skills (preferably on patients), discussing the competencies with

peer teachers and clinical instructors, practicing alone and with others, and then demonstrating proficiency to a peer teacher.

4. Demonstrate your proficiency to an ACI.

APPROVED BY
(date and signature, and mode for didactic)

1. Bones

Didactic _____

Lab _____

Peer _____

ACI _____

2. Articulations

Didactic _____

Lab _____

Peer _____

ACI _____

3. Ligaments

Didactic _____

Lab _____

Peer _____

ACI _____

4. Muscles

Didactic _____

Lab _____

Peer _____

ACI _____

5. Other structures

Didactic _____

Lab _____

Peer _____

ACI _____

6. History

Didactic _____

Lab _____

Peer _____

ACI _____

7. Special tests
Tibiofemoral alignment

Didactic _____

Lab _____

Peer _____

ACI _____

Patellar alignment

Didactic _____

Lab _____

Peer _____

ACI _____

Patellar glide, tilt, and rotation

Didactic _____

Lab _____

Peer _____

ACI _____

Valgus stress test

Didactic _____

Lab _____

Peer _____

ACI _____

Varus stress test

Didactic _____

Lab _____

Peer _____

ACI _____

Lachman's test

Didactic _____

Lab _____

Peer _____

ACI _____

Anterior drawer test

Didactic _____

Lab _____

Peer _____

ACI _____

Posterior drawer test

Didactic _____

Lab _____

Peer _____

ACI _____

Slocum test

Didactic _____

Lab _____

Peer _____

ACI _____

Bounce home test

Didactic _____

Lab _____

Peer _____

ACI _____

Godfrey 90/90 test

Didactic _____

Lab _____

Peer _____

ACI _____

Posterior sag (profile) sign

Didactic _____

Lab _____

Peer _____

ACI _____

Hughston's test

Didactic _____

Lab _____

Peer _____

ACI _____

Lateral pivot shift

Didactic _____

Lab _____

Peer _____

ACI _____

McMurray test

Didactic _____

Lab _____

Peer _____

ACI _____

Apley's compression and distraction test

Didactic _____

Lab _____

Peer _____

ACI _____

Thessaly test

Didactic _____

Lab _____

Peer _____

ACI _____

Patellar apprehension test

Didactic _____

Lab _____

Peer _____

ACI _____

Sweep test

Didactic _____

Lab _____

Peer _____

ACI _____

Ballottable patella

Didactic _____

Lab _____

Peer _____

ACI _____

8-14. Complete competencies 8 through 14 for the following injuries or conditions in list G:

Torn medial meniscus

Didactic _____

Lab _____

Peer _____

ACI _____

Torn lateral meniscus

Didactic _____

Lab _____

Peer _____

ACI _____

ACL sprain

Didactic _____

Lab _____

Peer _____

ACI _____

PCL sprain

Didactic _____

Lab _____

Peer _____

ACI _____

MCL sprain—superficial

Didactic _____

Lab _____

Peer _____

ACI _____

MCL sprain—deep

Didactic _____

Lab _____

Peer _____

ACI _____

LCL sprain

Didactic _____

Lab _____

Peer _____

ACI _____

AMRI

Didactic _____

Lab _____

Peer _____

ACI _____

ALRI

Didactic _____

Lab _____

Peer _____

ACI _____

Bursitis

Didactic _____

Lab _____

Peer _____

ACI _____

Capsular sprain

Didactic _____

Lab _____

Peer _____

ACI _____

Contused vastus medialis

Didactic _____

Lab _____

Peer _____

ACI _____

Patellofemoral joint pain

Didactic _____

Lab _____

Peer _____

ACI _____

Patellar tendinitis

Didactic _____

Lab _____

Peer _____

ACI _____

Patellar tendinosis

Didactic _____

Lab _____

Peer _____

ACI _____

Patellar tenosynovitis

Didactic _____

Lab _____

Peer _____

ACI _____

Fractured patella

Didactic _____

Lab _____

Peer _____

ACI _____

Baker's cyst

Didactic _____

Lab _____

Peer _____

ACI _____

Synovial plica

Didactic _____

Lab _____

Peer _____

ACI _____

Hyperextended knee

Didactic _____

Lab _____

Peer _____

ACI _____

Osgood-Schlatter disease

Didactic _____

Lab _____

Peer _____

ACI _____

Iliotibial band syndrome

Didactic _____

Lab _____

Peer _____

ACI _____

Distal hamstring strain

Didactic _____

Lab _____

Peer _____

ACI _____

Chondromalacia patella

Didactic _____

Lab _____

Peer _____

ACI _____

Patellar dislocation and subluxation

Didactic _____

Lab _____

Peer _____

ACI _____

Fat pad contusion

Didactic _____

Lab _____

Peer _____

ACI _____

Fracture

Didactic _____

Lab _____

Peer _____

ACI _____

Osteochondritis dissecans

Didactic _____

Lab _____

Peer _____

ACI _____

Patellar tendon rupture

Didactic _____

Lab _____

Peer _____

ACI _____

Peroneal nerve contusion or palsy

Didactic _____

Lab _____

Peer _____

ACI _____

Tendinitis

Didactic _____

Lab _____

Peer _____

ACI _____

Tibial torsion

Didactic _____

Lab _____

Peer _____

ACI _____

COMMENTS

_____

_____

_____

_____

_____

_____

_____

Thigh, Hip, and Pelvic Injury Assessment and Diagnosis

Objective

Develop and demonstrate the skills necessary to evaluate thigh, hip, and pelvic injuries.

NATA Athletic Training Educational Competencies embedded in this module: AC-C6, DI-C6, DI-C7, DI-C10, DI-C12, DI-C13, DI-C15, DI-C16, DI-C17, DI-P1, DI-P2, DI-P4, DI-P5, DI-P6, DI-P7, DI-P8, DI-P10, DI-CP1

Anatomy and Conditions for This Module

A. Bones and Prominent Bony Features

- Femur
  - Condyles
  - Epicondyles
- Tibia
  - Medial condyle
  - Lateral condyle
  - Gerdy's tubercle
  - Patellar tubercle
- Fibula
  - Head
  - Proximal shaft
- Patella
- Ilium
  - Crest
  - Tubercle
  - Anterior inferior spine
  - Anterior superior spine
  - Posterior superior spine
- Pubis
  - Ramus
  - Tubercle
- Ischium
  - Tubercle or tuberosity
  - Obturator foramen
- Femur
  - Greater trochanter
  - Lesser trochanter
  - Linea aspera
  - Fovea capitis
- Spine
  - Lumbar vertebrae
  - Sacrum
  - Coccyx

B. Articulations

- Medial tibiofemoral
- Lateral tibiofemoral
- Patellotibial
- Sacroiliac
- Lumbosacral
- Hip
- Pubic symphysis

C. Ligaments

- Inguinal
- Supraspinous
- Interspinous
- Intertransverse
- Longitudinal (posterior and anterior)
- Iliofemoral
- Iliotibial band

D. Muscles

- Biceps femoris (long and short heads)
- Semitendinosus
- Semimembranosus
- Rectus femoris
- Vastus medialis
- Vastus intermedius
- Vastus lateralis
- Sartorius
- Hip adductor group
- Tensor fasciae latae
- Iliotibial band
- Gracilis
- Gluteus maximus
- Gluteus medius
- Gluteus minimus
- Iliopsoas
- Psoas major
- Iliacus
- Adductor brevis
- Adductor magnus
- Latissimus dorsi
- Paraspinal
- External obliques

- Internal obliques
- Transverse abdominis

E. Other Structures

- Femoral nerve
- Sciatic nerve
- Lateral cutaneous nerve
- Trochanteric bursae
- Iliopsoas bursae
- Male genitalia
- Female genitalia
- Anus
- Bladder
- Bowels

F. Special Tests

- Leg length discrepancies
- Patrick's (FABER) test
- Fulcrum test
- Gaenslen's test
- Pelvic compression (squish) or distraction (gapping) test
- Sacroiliac joint fixation test
- Femoral nerve traction test
- Trendelenburg's test
- Piriformis test
- Thomas or Kendall test
- Rectus femoris contracture test
- Ober's test
- Noble's test
- Hip scouring test

G. Injuries and Conditions

- Quadriceps contusion
- Quadriceps strain
- Hamstring strain
- Femoral fracture
- Myositis ossificans
- Patellar tendon rupture
- Snapping hip
- Lateral hip pain
- Hip retroversion
- Hip anteversion
- Hip sprain
- Contused iliac crest (hip pointer)
- Dislocated hip

- Proximal hamstring strain
- Proximal sartorius strain
- Hip flexor strain
- Hip adductor strain
- Gluteal strain
- Hernia
- Contused genitalia
- Spermatic cord torsion
- Traumatic hydrocele of the tunica vaginalis
- Femur fracture
- Pelvic fracture
- Trochanteric bursitis
- Iliopsoas bursitis
- Sacroiliac dysfunction
- Legg-Calvé-Perthes disease
- Apophysitis
- Slipped capital femoral epiphysis
- Dislocation or subluxation
- Stress fracture
- Osteitis pubis
- Athletic pubalgia
- Bursitis
- Piriformis syndrome
- Iliotibial band syndrome
- Contusion
- Tendinitis
- Arthritis
- Avascular necrosis—femoral head

Competencies

Note: All procedures must be performed.

Anatomical Review and Assessment of Structural Integrity

1. Name and palpate each bone and bony structure in list A. Tell what differences you would expect to feel if the bone were fractured.

2. Palpate or draw the joint line for each articulation in list B. Then perform active and passive joint ROM tests using both qualitative and quantitative techniques (e.g., tape measure, goniometer, and inclinometer). Record the results of these tests using accepted forms and procedures.

3. Using surface anatomy, palpate or draw the origins and course of each ligament in list C.

4. Using surface anatomy, palpate the origin, insertion, and course of each muscle in list D. Also, tell the major function of each muscle.

5. Using surface anatomy, palpate each structure in list E.

Injury Assessment

6. Obtain the medical history of an athlete with a suspected hip and pelvis injury.

7. Demonstrate proper administration and interpretation of the special tests in list F.

8. Demonstrate how you would observe and identify the clinical signs and symptoms associated with the injuries and conditions in list G.

9. Explain and demonstrate the mechanisms by which each injury in list G occurs. Name the three sports in which each injury is most likely to occur and explain any differences among the injury occurrences and mechanisms in those sports.

10. Demonstrate appropriate sensory, circulatory, and neurological tests for the injuries in list G.

11. Palpate and assess the integrity of the bones and soft tissues associated with each injury in list G.

12. Perform special tests to assess the integrity of the joints involved in each injury in list G and explain how you would interpret these tests.

13. Demonstrate the use of manual muscle testing and other tests as appropriate to assess the flexibility and strength of the muscles associated with each injury in list G.

14. Demonstrate functional and activity-specific tests to determine the integrity of each structure involved in each injury in list G.

Proficiency Demonstration

1. Develop appropriate subject knowledge through coursework (C), verbal conversation (V), quizzes (Q), worksheets (W), or other approved activities (O).

2. Practice and reinforce the skills in clinical skills and laboratory courses.

3. Refine your skills by observing peer teachers and clinical instructors as they perform the skills (preferably on patients), discussing the competencies with peer teachers and clinical instructors, practicing alone and with others, and then demonstrating proficiency to a peer teacher.

4. Demonstrate your proficiency to an ACI.

APPROVED BY
(date and signature, and mode for didactic)

1. Bones
   Didactic _____
   Lab _____
   Peer _____
   ACI _____

2. Articulations
   Didactic _____
   Lab _____
   Peer _____
   ACI _____

3. Ligaments
   Didactic _____
   Lab _____
   Peer _____
   ACI _____

4. Muscles
   Didactic _____
   Lab _____
   Peer _____
   ACI _____

5. Other structures
   Didactic _____
   Lab _____
   Peer _____
   ACI _____

6. History
   Didactic _____
   Lab _____
   Peer _____
   ACI _____

7. Special tests
   Leg length discrepancies
   Didactic _____
   Lab _____
   Peer _____
   ACI _____

Patrick's (FABER) test

Didactic _____

Lab _____

Peer _____

ACI _____

Fulcrum test

Didactic _____

Lab _____

Peer _____

ACI _____

Gaenslen's test

Didactic _____

Lab _____

Peer _____

ACI _____

Pelvic compression (squish) or distraction (gapping) test

Didactic _____

Lab _____

Peer _____

ACI _____

Sacroiliac joint fixation test

Didactic _____

Lab _____

Peer _____

ACI _____

Femoral nerve traction test

Didactic _____

Lab _____

Peer _____

ACI _____

Trendelenburg's test

Didactic _____

Lab _____

Peer _____

ACI _____

Piriformis test

Didactic _____

Lab _____

Peer _____

ACI _____

Thomas or Kendall test

Didactic _____

Lab _____

Peer _____

ACI _____

Ober's test

Didactic _____

Lab _____

Peer _____

ACI _____

Noble's test

Didactic _____

Lab _____

Peer _____

ACI _____

Hip scouring test

Didactic _____

Lab _____

Peer _____

ACI _____

8-14. Complete competencies 8 through 14 for the injuries or conditions in list G:

Quadriceps contusion

Didactic _____

Lab _____

Peer _____

ACI _____

Quadriceps strain

Didactic _____

Lab _____

Peer _____

ACI _____

Hamstring strain

Didactic _____

Lab _____

Peer _____

ACI _____

Femoral fracture

Didactic _____

Lab _____

Peer _____

ACI _____

Myositis ossificans

Didactic _____

Lab _____

Peer _____

ACI _____

Patellar tendon rupture

Didactic _____

Lab _____

Peer _____

ACI _____

Snapping hip

Didactic _____

Lab _____

Peer _____

ACI _____

Lateral hip pain

Didactic _____

Lab _____

Peer _____

ACI _____

Hip retroversion

Didactic _____

Lab _____

Peer _____

ACI _____

Hip anteversion

Didactic _____

Lab _____

Peer _____

ACI _____

Hip sprain

Didactic _____

Lab _____

Peer _____

ACI _____

Contused iliac crest

Didactic _____

Lab _____

Peer _____

ACI _____

Dislocated hip

Didactic _____

Lab _____

Peer _____

ACI _____

Proximal hamstring strain

Didactic _____

Lab _____

Peer _____

ACI _____

Proximal sartorius strain

Didactic _____

Lab _____

Peer _____

ACI _____

Hip flexor strain

Didactic _____

Lab _____

Peer _____

ACI _____

Hip adductor strain

Didactic _____

Lab _____

Peer _____

ACI _____

Gluteal strain

Didactic _____

Lab _____

Peer _____

ACI _____

Hernia

Didactic _____

Lab _____

Peer _____

ACI _____

Contused genitalia

Didactic _____

Lab _____

Peer _____

ACI _____

Spermatic cord torsion

Didactic _____

Lab _____

Peer _____

ACI _____

Traumatic hydrocele of the tunica vaginalis

Didactic _____

Lab _____

Peer _____

ACI _____

Femur fracture

Didactic _____

Lab _____

Peer _____

ACI _____

Pelvic fracture

Didactic _____

Lab _____

Peer _____

ACI _____

Trochanteric bursitis

Didactic _____

Lab _____

Peer _____

ACI _____

Iliopsoas bursitis

Didactic _____

Lab _____

Peer _____

ACI _____

Sacroiliac dysfunction

Didactic _____

Lab _____

Peer _____

ACI _____

Legg-Calvé-Perthes disease

Didactic _____

Lab _____

Peer _____

ACI _____

Apophysitis

Didactic _____

Lab _____

Peer _____

ACI _____

Slipped capital femoral epiphysis

Didactic _____

Lab _____

Peer _____

ACI _____

Dislocation or subluxation

Didactic _____

Lab _____

Peer _____

ACI _____

Stress fracture

Didactic _____

Lab _____

Peer _____

ACI _____

Osteitis pubis

Didactic _____

Lab _____

Peer _____

ACI _____

Athletic pubalgia

Didactic _____

Lab _____

Peer _____

ACI _____

Bursitis

Didactic _____

Lab _____

Peer _____

ACI _____

Piriformis syndrome

Didactic _____

Lab _____

Peer _____

ACI _____

Iliotibial band syndrome

Didactic _____

Lab _____

Peer _____

ACI _____

Contusion

Didactic _____

Lab _____

Peer _____

ACI _____

Tendinitis

Didactic _____

Lab _____

Peer _____

ACI _____

Arthritis

Didactic _____

Lab _____

Peer _____

ACI _____

Avascular necrosis—femoral head

Didactic _____

Lab _____

Peer _____

ACI _____

COMMENTS

_____

_____

_____

_____

_____

_____

_____

Thorax and Lumbar Spine Injury Assessment and Diagnosis

Objective

Develop and demonstrate the skills necessary to evaluate low back injuries.

NATA Athletic Training Educational Competencies embedded in this module: AC-C6, AC-C22, DI-C6, DI-C7, DI-C8, DI-C9, DI-C10, DI-C11, DI-C12, DI-C13, DI-C15, DI-C16, DI-C17, DI-P1, DI-P2, DI-P3, DI-P4, DI-P5, DI-P6, DI-P7, DI-P8, DI-P9, DI-P10, DI-CP1

Anatomy and Conditions for This Module

A. Bones and Prominent Bony Features

- Ilium
  - Crest
  - Tubercle
  - Anterior inferior spine
  - Anterior superior spine
  - Posterior superior spine
- Pubis
  - Tubercle
  - Pubic symphysis
- Ischium
  - Tubercle or tuberosity
  - Obturator foramen
- Femur
  - Greater trochanter
  - Lesser trochanter
  - Head of femur
  - Neck of femur
- Spine
  - Thoracic vertebrae
  - Lumbar vertebrae
  - Spinous processes
  - Sacrum
  - Coccyx

B. Articulations

- Sacroiliac
- Lumbosacral
- Hip
- Thoracic intervertebral
- Lumbar intervertebral
- Costothoracic

C. Ligaments

- Supraspinous
- Interspinous
- Intertransverse
- Longitudinal (posterior and anterior)

D. Muscles

- Rhomboids
- Lower trapezius
- Rectus abdominis
- External oblique
- Internal oblique
- Transverse abdominis
- Gluteus maximus
- Gluteus medius
- Gluteus minimus
- Tensor fasciae latae
- Hamstrings
- Iliopsoas
- Psoas major
- Iliacus
- Paraspinal

E. Other Structures

- Bladder
- Liver
- Spleen
- Kidneys
- Pancreas
- Gall bladder
- Stomach
- Small intestine
- Large intestine

F. Special Tests

- Spinal posture (kyphosis and lordosis)
- Leg length discrepancies
- Valsalva maneuver
- Lasegue's test
- Well straight-leg test
- Milgram's test
- Sitting root test
- Quadrant (facet joint) test

- Kernig's and Brudzinski's signs
- Bowstring test
- Hoover's sign
- Stork standing (spondylolisthesis) test
- Spring test
- Lower-extremity neurological evaluation (lower-quarter screen)

G. Injuries and Conditions

- Café au lait macules (spots)
- Dislocation or subluxation
- Thoracic sprain or strain
- Lumbar sprain or strain
- Lumbosacral sprain or strain
- Contusion
- Sacroiliac dysfunction
- Intervertebral disc pathology
- Facet syndrome
- Nerve root compression
- Stenosis
- Step deformity
- Sciatica
- Spondylolysis
- Spondylolisthesis
- Spondylitis
- Scoliosis
- Transverse spinous process fracture
- Spina bifida occulta

Competencies

Note: All procedures must be performed.

Anatomical Review and Assessment of Structural Integrity

1. Name and palpate each bone and bony structure in list A. Tell what differences you would expect to feel if the bone were fractured.

2. Palpate or draw the joint line for each articulation in list B. Then perform active and passive joint ROM tests using both qualitative and quantitative techniques (e.g., tape measure, goniometer, and inclinometer). Record the results of these tests using accepted forms and procedures.

3. Using surface anatomy, palpate or draw the origins and course of each ligament in list C.

4. Using surface anatomy, palpate the origin, insertion, and course of each muscle in list D. Also, tell the major function of each muscle.

5. Using surface anatomy, palpate each structure in list E.

Injury Assessment

6. Obtain the medical history of an athlete with a suspected thoracic or lumbar spine injury.

7. Demonstrate proper administration and interpretation of the special tests in list F.

8. Demonstrate how you would observe and identify the clinical signs and symptoms associated with the injuries and conditions in list G.

9. Explain and demonstrate the mechanisms by which each injury in list G occurs. Name the three sports in which each injury is most likely to occur and explain any differences among the injury occurrences and mechanisms in those sports.

10. Demonstrate appropriate sensory, circulatory, and neurological tests for the injuries in list G.

11. Palpate and assess the integrity of the bones and soft tissues associated with each injury in list G.

12. Perform special tests to assess the integrity of the joints involved in each injury in list G and explain how you would interpret these tests.

13. Demonstrate the use of manual muscle testing and other tests as appropriate to assess the flexibility and strength of the muscles associated with each injury in list G.

14. Demonstrate functional and activity-specific tests to determine the integrity of each structure involved in each injury in list G.

Proficiency Demonstration

1. Develop appropriate subject knowledge through coursework (C), verbal conversation (V), quizzes (Q), worksheets (W), or other approved activities (O).

2. Practice and reinforce the skills in clinical skills and laboratory courses.

3. Refine your skills by observing peer teachers and clinical instructors as they perform the skills (preferably on patients), discussing the competencies with peer teachers and clinical instructors, practicing alone and with others, and then demonstrating proficiency to a peer teacher.

4. Demonstrate your proficiency to an ACI.

APPROVED BY
(date and signature, and mode for didactic)

1. Bones
   Didactic _____
   Lab _____
   Peer _____
   ACI _____

2. Articulations
   Didactic _____
   Lab _____
   Peer _____
   ACI _____

3. Ligaments
   Didactic _____
   Lab _____
   Peer _____
   ACI _____

4. Muscles
   Didactic _____
   Lab _____
   Peer _____
   ACI _____

5. Other structures
   Didactic _____
   Lab _____
   Peer _____
   ACI _____

6. History
   Didactic _____
   Lab _____
   Peer _____
   ACI _____

7. Special tests
   Spinal posture
   Didactic _____
   Lab _____
   Peer _____
   ACI _____

Leg length discrepancies
Didactic _____
Lab _____
Peer _____
ACI _____

Valsalva maneuver
Didactic _____
Lab _____
Peer _____
ACI _____

Lasegue's test
Didactic _____
Lab _____
Peer _____
ACI _____

Well straight-leg test
Didactic _____
Lab _____
Peer _____
ACI _____

Milgram's test
Didactic _____
Lab _____
Peer _____
ACI _____

Sitting root test
Didactic _____
Lab _____
Peer _____
ACI _____

Quadrant (facet joint) test
Didactic _____
Lab _____
Peer _____
ACI _____

Kernig and Brudzinski's signs

Didactic _____

Lab _____

Peer _____

ACI _____

Bowstring test

Didactic _____

Lab _____

Peer _____

ACI _____

Hoover's sign

Didactic _____

Lab _____

Peer _____

ACI _____

Stork standing (spondylolisthesis) test

Didactic _____

Lab _____

Peer _____

ACI _____

Spring test

Didactic _____

Lab _____

Peer _____

ACI _____

Lower-extremity neurological evaluation

Didactic _____

Lab _____

Peer _____

ACI _____

8-14. Complete competencies 8 through 14 for the injuries or conditions in list G:

Café au lait macules

Didactic _____

Lab _____

Peer _____

ACI _____

Dislocation or subluxation

Didactic _____

Lab _____

Peer _____

ACI _____

Thoracic sprain or strain

Didactic _____

Lab _____

Peer _____

ACI _____

Lumbar sprain or strain

Didactic _____

Lab _____

Peer _____

ACI _____

Lumbosacral sprain or strain

Didactic _____

Lab _____

Peer _____

ACI _____

Contusion

Didactic _____

Lab _____

Peer _____

ACI _____

Sacroiliac dysfunction

Didactic _____

Lab _____

Peer _____

ACI _____

Intervertebral disc pathology

Didactic _____

Lab _____

Peer _____

ACI _____

Facet syndrome

Didactic _____

Lab _____

Peer _____

ACI _____

Nerve root compression

Didactic _____

Lab _____

Peer _____

ACI _____

Stenosis

Didactic _____

Lab _____

Peer _____

ACI _____

Step deformity

Didactic _____

Lab _____

Peer _____

ACI _____

Sciatica

Didactic _____

Lab _____

Peer _____

ACI _____

Spondylolysis

Didactic _____

Lab _____

Peer _____

ACI _____

Spondylolisthesis

Didactic _____

Lab _____

Peer _____

ACI _____

Spondylitis

Didactic _____

Lab _____

Peer _____

ACI _____

Scoliosis

Didactic _____

Lab _____

Peer _____

ACI _____

Transverse spinous process fracture

Didactic _____

Lab _____

Peer _____

ACI _____

Spina bifida occulta

Didactic _____

Lab _____

Peer _____

ACI _____

COMMENTS

_____

_____

_____

_____

_____

_____

_____

_____

Thorax and Abdominal Injury Assessment and Diagnosis

Objective

Develop and demonstrate the skills necessary to evaluate thorax and abdominal injuries.

NATA Athletic Training Educational Competencies embedded in this module: DI-C6, DI-C7, DI-C10, DI-C13, DI-C16, DI-C17, DI-P1, DI-P2, DI-P3, DI-P4, DI-P7, DI-P8, DI-P10, DI-CP1, MC-C3, MC-C7, MC-C8, MC-P1, MC-P2, MC-P3, MC-P4, MC-CP1

Anatomy and Conditions for This Module

A. Bones and Prominent Bony Features

- Ilium
  - Crest
  - Tubercle
  - Anterior inferior spine
  - Anterior superior spine
  - Posterior superior spine
- Spine
  - Thoracic vertebrae
  - Lumbar vertebrae
  - Spinous processes
- Rib cage
  - Ribs
  - Floating ribs
  - Costal cartilage
- Sternum
  - Manubrium
  - Body
  - Xiphoid process

B. Articulations

- Sternoclavicular
- Costosternal
- Costovertebral
- Costochondral

C. Muscles

- Rectus abdominis
- Obliques
- Transverse abdominis
- Latissimus dorsi
- Erector spinae
- Quadratus lumborum
- Intercostals
- Diaphragm

D. Other Structures

- Phrenic nerve
- Heart
- Lungs
- Pancreas
- Liver
- Spleen
- Kidneys
- Stomach
- Intestine
- Gallbladder
- Urinary bladder

E. Special Tests

- Auscultation of heart, lungs, and abdomen
  - Abdominal percussion
  - Rebound tenderness test
- Blood pressure, pulse, spirometry
  - Rib compression test
  - Sternoclavicular joint stress test
- Kehr's sign
  - Beevor's sign
  - McBurney's point tenderness

F. Injuries and Conditions

- Abdominal muscular strain
- Rectus abdominis contusion
- Spleen rupture
- Kidney contusion
- Stitch in the side
- Solar plexus trauma
- Sternoclavicular separation
- Sternal fracture
- Rib fracture
- Rib contusion
- Costochondral dislocation
- Pneumothorax
- Hemothorax

Competencies

Note: All procedures must be performed.

Anatomical Review and Assessment of Structural Integrity

1. Name and palpate each bone and bony structures in list A. Tell what differences you would expect to feel if the bone were fractured.

2. Palpate or draw the joint line for each articulation in list B. Then perform active and passive joint ROM tests using both qualitative and quantitative techniques (e.g., tape measure, goniometer, and inclinometer). Record the results of these tests using accepted forms and procedures.

3. Using surface anatomy, palpate the origin, insertion, and course of each muscle in list C. Also, tell the major function of each muscle.

4. Using surface anatomy, palpate each structure in list D.

Injury Assessment and Diagnosis

5. Obtain the medical history of an athlete with a suspected thorax or abdominal injury.

6. Demonstrate how you would observe and identify the clinical signs and symptoms associated with the injuries and conditions in list F.

7. Explain and demonstrate the mechanisms by which each injury in list F occurs. Name the three sports in which each injury is most likely to occur and explain any differences among the injury occurrences and mechanisms in those sports.

8. Demonstrate appropriate sensory, circulatory, and neurological tests for the injuries in list F.

9. Palpate and assess the integrity of the bones and soft tissues associated with each injury in list F.

10. Perform special tests to assess the integrity of the joints involved in each injury in list F and explain how you would interpret these tests.

11. Demonstrate the use of manual muscle testing and other tests as appropriate to assess the flexibility and strength of the muscles associated with each injury in list F.

12. Demonstrate functional and activity-specific tests to determine the integrity of each structure involved in each injury in list E.

13. Perform special tests.

Proficiency Demonstration

1. Develop appropriate subject knowledge through coursework (C), verbal conversation (V), quizzes (Q), worksheets (W), or other approved activities (O).

2. Practice and reinforce the skills in clinical skills and laboratory courses.

3. Refine your skills by observing peer teachers and clinical instructors as they perform the skills (preferably on patients), discussing the competencies with peer teachers and clinical instructors, practicing alone and with others, and then demonstrating proficiency to a peer teacher.

4. Demonstrate your proficiency to an ACI.

APPROVED BY
(date and signature, and mode for didactic)

1. Bones

    Didactic _____

    Lab _____

    Peer _____

    ACI _____

2. Articulations

    Didactic _____

    Lab _____

    Peer _____

    ACI _____

3. Muscles

    Didactic _____

    Lab _____

    Peer _____

    ACI _____

4. Other structures

    Didactic _____

    Lab _____

    Peer _____

    ACI _____

5. History

    Didactic _____

    Lab _____

    Peer _____

    ACI _____

6. Special tests

Auscultation of heart, lungs, and abdomen

Didactic _____

Lab _____

Peer _____

ACI _____

Abdominal percussion

Didactic _____

Lab _____

Peer _____

ACI _____

Rebound tenderness test

Didactic _____

Lab _____

Peer _____

ACI _____

Blood pressure, pulse, spirometry

Didactic _____

Lab _____

Peer _____

ACI _____

Rib compression test

Didactic _____

Lab _____

Peer _____

ACI _____

Sternoclavicular joint stress test

Didactic _____

Lab _____

Peer _____

ACI _____

Kehr's sign

Didactic _____

Lab _____

Peer _____

ACI _____

Beevor's sign

Didactic _____

Lab _____

Peer _____

ACI _____

McBurney's point tenderness

Didactic _____

Lab _____

Peer _____

ACI _____

7-13. Complete competencies 7 through 13 for the injuries or conditions in list F:

Abdominal strain

Didactic _____

Lab _____

Peer _____

ACI _____

Rectus abdominis contusion

Didactic _____

Lab _____

Peer _____

ACI _____

Spleen rupture

Didactic _____

Lab _____

Peer _____

ACI _____

Kidney contusion

Didactic _____

Lab _____

Peer _____

ACI _____

Stitch in the side

Didactic _____

Lab _____

Peer _____

ACI _____

Solar plexus trauma

Didactic _____

Lab _____

Peer _____

ACI _____

Sternoclavicular separation

Didactic _____

Lab _____

Peer _____

ACI _____

Sternal fracture

Didactic _____

Lab _____

Peer _____

ACI _____

Rib fracture

Didactic _____

Lab _____

Peer _____

ACI _____

Rib contusion

Didactic _____

Lab _____

Peer _____

ACI _____

Costochondral dislocation

Didactic _____

Lab _____

Peer _____

ACI _____

Pneumothorax

Didactic _____

Lab _____

Peer _____

ACI _____

Hemothorax

Didactic _____

Lab _____

Peer _____

ACI _____

COMMENTS

_____

_____

_____

_____

_____

Shoulder Injury Assessment and Diagnosis

Objective

Develop and demonstrate the skills necessary to evaluate shoulder injuries.

NATA Athletic Training Educational Competencies embedded in this module: AC-C6, DI-C6, DI-C7, DI-C10, DI-C12, DI-C13, DI-C15, DI-C16, DI-C17, DI-P1, DI-P2, DI-P4, DI-P5, DI-P6, DI-P7, DI-P8, DI-P10, DI-CP1

Anatomy and Conditions for This Module

A. Bones and Prominent Bony Features

- Ribs
- Sternum
  - Manubrium
  - Body
- Clavicle
- Scapula
  - Suprapatellar fossa
  - Spine
  - Infrapatellar fossa
  - Acromion process
  - Coracoid process
  - Medial border
  - Lateral border
  - Inferior angle
- Humerus
  - Greater trochanter
  - Lesser trochanter
  - Bicipital groove

B. Articulations

- Glenohumeral
- Acromioclavicular
- Coracoclavicular
- Sternoclavicular
- Scapulothoracic

C. Ligaments

- Glenohumeral
  - Anterior
  - Middle
  - Posterior
- Acromioclavicular
- Coracoclavicular
- Coracoacromial
- Sternoclavicular

D. Muscles

- Biceps (both heads)
- Triceps (all three heads)
- Deltoid (all three portions)
- Pectoralis major
- Pectoralis minor
- Teres major
- Teres minor
- Latissimus dorsi
- Supraspinatus
- Infraspinatus
- Subscapularis
- Trapezius
- Rhomboids
- Levator scapulae
- Serratus anterior
- Subclavius

E. Other Structures

- Subacromial bursa
- Subdeltoid bursa
- Brachial plexus
- Axillary nerve

F. Special Tests

- Symmetry, efficiency of movement, scapulohumeral rhythm
- Apley scratch test
- Jerk (posterior stress) test
- Glenohumeral glide tests
- Jobe relocation test (Fowler's sign)
- Apprehension tests
- Clunk test
- Grind test
- Sulcus sign
- Acromioclavicular compression test
- Speed's test
- Drop arm test
- Empty can test
- Gerber liftoff test
- Crossover impingement test
- Hawkins-Kennedy impingement test
- O'Brien's (active compression) test

- Brachial plexus stretch test
- Neer impingement test
- Pectoralis major contracture test
- Yergason's test
- Adson's maneuver

G. Injuries and Conditions

- Fracture
- Nerve injury
- Step deformity
- Scapular winging
- Sternoclavicular sprain or dislocation
- Clavicular fracture
- Acromioclavicular instability
- Glenohumeral instability
- Recurrent glenohumeral dislocation
- Subacromial impingement
- Rotator cuff strain
- Subacromial bursitis
- Tenosynovitis and tendinitis
- Bicipital subluxation
- Thoracic outlet syndrome
- Epiphyseal fracture
- Throwing injuries
- Sprengel's deformity

Competencies

Note: All procedures must be performed.

Anatomical Review and Assessment of Structural Integrity

1. Name and palpate each bone and bony structures in list A. Tell what differences you would expect to feel if the bone were fractured.

2. Palpate or draw the joint line for each articulation in list B. Then perform active and passive joint ROM tests using both qualitative and quantitative techniques (e.g., tape measure, goniometer, and inclinometer). Record the results of these tests using accepted forms and procedures.

3. Using surface anatomy, palpate or draw the origins and course of each ligament in list C.

4. Using surface anatomy, palpate the origin, insertion, and course of each muscle in list D. Also, tell the major function of each muscle.

5. Using surface anatomy, palpate each structure in list E.

Injury Assessment

6. Obtain the medical history of an athlete with a suspected shoulder injury.

7. Demonstrate proper administration and interpretation of the special tests in list F.

8. Demonstrate how you would observe and identify the clinical signs and symptoms associated with the injuries and conditions in list G.

9. Explain and demonstrate the mechanisms by which each injury in list G occurs. Name the three sports in which each injury is most likely to occur and explain any differences among the injury occurrences and mechanisms in those sports.

10. Demonstrate appropriate sensory, circulatory, and neurological tests for the injuries in list G.

11. Palpate and assess the integrity of the bones and soft tissues associated with each injury in list G.

12. Perform special tests to assess the integrity of the joints involved in each injury in list G and explain how you would interpret these tests.

13. Demonstrate the use of manual muscle testing and other tests as appropriate to assess the flexibility and strength of the muscles associated with each injury in list G.

14. Demonstrate functional and activity-specific tests to determine the integrity of each structure involved in each injury in list G.

Proficiency Demonstration

1. Develop appropriate subject knowledge through coursework (C), verbal conversation (V), quizzes (Q), worksheets (W), or other approved activities (O).

2. Practice and reinforce the skills in clinical skills and laboratory courses.

3. Refine your skills by observing peer teachers and clinical instructors as they perform the skills (preferably on patients), discussing the competencies with peer teachers and clinical instructors, practicing alone and with others, and then demonstrating proficiency to a peer teacher.

4. Demonstrate your proficiency to an ACI.

APPROVED BY
(date and signature, and mode for didactic)

1. Bones
   Didactic _____
   Lab _____
   Peer _____
   ACI _____

2. Articulations
   Didactic _____
   Lab _____
   Peer _____
   ACI _____

3. Ligaments
   Didactic _____
   Lab _____
   Peer _____
   ACI _____

4. Muscles
   Didactic _____
   Lab _____
   Peer _____
   ACI _____

5. Other structures
   Didactic _____
   Lab _____
   Peer _____
   ACI _____

6. History
   Didactic _____
   Lab _____
   Peer _____
   ACI _____

7. Special tests

   Symmetry, efficiency of movement, scapulohumeral rhythm
   Didactic _____
   Lab _____
   Peer _____
   ACI _____

Apley scratch test
Didactic _____
Lab _____
Peer _____
ACI _____

Jerk (posterior stress) test
Didactic _____
Lab _____
Peer _____
ACI _____

Glenohumeral glide tests
Didactic _____
Lab _____
Peer _____
ACI _____

Jobe relocation test (Fowler's sign)
Didactic _____
Lab _____
Peer _____
ACI _____

Apprehension tests
Didactic _____
Lab _____
Peer _____
ACI _____

Clunk test
Didactic _____
Lab _____
Peer _____
ACI _____

Grind test
Didactic _____
Lab _____
Peer _____
ACI _____

Sulcus sign

Didactic _____

Lab _____

Peer _____

ACI _____

Acromioclavicular compression test

Didactic _____

Lab _____

Peer _____

ACI _____

Speed's test

Didactic _____

Lab _____

Peer _____

ACI _____

Drop arm test

Didactic _____

Lab _____

Peer _____

ACI _____

Empty can test

Didactic _____

Lab _____

Peer _____

ACI _____

Gerber liftoff test

Didactic _____

Lab _____

Peer _____

ACI _____

Crossover impingement test

Didactic _____

Lab _____

Peer _____

ACI _____

Hawkins-Kennedy impingement test

Didactic _____

Lab _____

Peer _____

ACI _____

O'Brien's (active compression) test

Didactic _____

Lab _____

Peer _____

ACI _____

Brachial plexus stretch test

Didactic _____

Lab _____

Peer _____

ACI _____

Neer impingement test

Didactic _____

Lab _____

Peer _____

ACI _____

Pectoralis major contracture test

Didactic _____

Lab _____

Peer _____

ACI _____

Yergason's test

Didactic _____

Lab _____

Peer _____

ACI _____

Adson's maneuver

Didactic _____

Lab _____

Peer _____

ACI _____

8-14. Complete competencies 8 through 14 for the injuries or conditions in list G:

Fracture

Didactic _____

Lab _____

Peer _____

ACI _____

Nerve injury

Didactic _____

Lab _____

Peer _____

ACI _____

Step deformity

Didactic _____

Lab _____

Peer _____

ACI _____

Scapular winging

Didactic _____

Lab _____

Peer _____

ACI _____

Sternoclavicular sprain or dislocation

Didactic _____

Lab _____

Peer _____

ACI _____

Clavicular fracture

Didactic _____

Lab _____

Peer _____

ACI _____

Acromioclavicular instability

Didactic _____

Lab _____

Peer _____

ACI _____

Glenohumeral instability

Didactic _____

Lab _____

Peer _____

ACI _____

Recurrent glenohumeral dislocation

Didactic _____

Lab _____

Peer _____

ACI _____

Subacromial impingement

Didactic _____

Lab _____

Peer _____

ACI _____

Rotator cuff strain

Didactic _____

Lab _____

Peer _____

ACI _____

Subacromial bursitis

Didactic _____

Lab _____

Peer _____

ACI _____

Tenosynovitis and tendinitis

Didactic _____

Lab _____

Peer _____

ACI _____

Bicipital subluxation

Didactic _____

Lab _____

Peer _____

ACI _____

Thoracic outlet syndrome

Didactic _____

Lab _____

Peer _____

ACI _____

Epiphyseal fracture

Didactic _____

Lab _____

Peer _____

ACI _____

Throwing injuries

Didactic _____

Lab _____

Peer _____

ACI _____

Sprengel's deformity

Didactic _____

Lab _____

Peer _____

ACI _____

COMMENTS

_____

_____

_____

_____

_____

_____

_____

_____

Arm and Elbow Injury Assessment and Diagnosis

Objective

Develop and demonstrate the skills necessary to evaluate arm and elbow injuries.

NATA Athletic Training Educational Competencies embedded in this module: AC-C6, DI-C6, DI-C7, DI-C10, DI-C12, DI-C13, DI-C15, DI-C16, DI-C17, DI-P1, DI-P2, DI-P4, DI-P5, DI-P6, DI-P7, DI-P8, DI-P10, DI-CP1

Anatomy and Conditions for This Module

A. Bones and Prominent Bony Features

- Humerus
  - Greater trochanter
  - Lesser trochanter
  - Bicipital groove
  - Capitulum
  - Olecranon fossa
  - Trochlea
- Ulna
  - Olecranon process
  - Coronoid process
  - Trochlea notch
  - Radial notch
  - Interosseous border
- Radius
  - Head
  - Interosseous border
  - Ulnar notch

B. Articulations

- Radiohumeral
- Ulnohumeral
- Proximal radioulnar

C. Ligaments

- Annular
- Ulnar collateral
- Radial collateral
- Interosseous

D. Muscles

- Biceps (both heads)
- Triceps (all three heads)
- Coracobrachialis
- Brachialis
- Brachioradialis
- Anconeus
- Pronator teres
- Pronator quadratus
- Flexor carpi radialis
- Flexor carpi ulnaris
- Extensor digitorum
- Supinator

E. Other Structures

- Median nerve
- Radial nerve
- Ulnar nerve
- Radial artery
- Olecranon bursa
- Radiohumeral bursa

F. Special Tests

- Symmetry, carrying angle (cubital valgus and varus), efficiency of movement
- Valgus stress test
- Varus stress test
- Moving valgus stress test
- Cozen's (tennis elbow) test
- Resistive tennis elbow test
- Passive tennis elbow test
- Medial epicondylitis (golfer's elbow) test
- Hyperextension test
- Tinel's sign

G. Injuries and Conditions

- Bicipital strain
- Humeral fracture
- Epiphyseal fracture
- Humeral contusion
- Humeral exostoses
- Supracondylar fracture
- Olecranon bursitis
- Medial elbow strain
- Medial collateral ligament sprain
- Elbow hyperextension
- Elbow dislocation
- Elbow fracture
- Radial nerve injury
- Throwing injury

- Medial epicondylitis
- Lateral epicondylitis
- Forearm contusion
- Radial head fracture
- Forearm splint
- Dislocation or subluxation
- Pronator teres syndrome
- Nerve injury
- Bursitis
- Osteochondritis dissecans

Competencies

Note: All procedures must be performed.

Anatomical Review and Assessment of Structural Integrity

1. Name and palpate each bone and bony structure in list A. Tell what differences you would expect to feel if the bone were fractured.

2. Palpate or draw the joint line for each articulation in list B. Then perform active and passive joint ROM tests using both qualitative and quantitative techniques (e.g., tape measure, goniometer, and inclinometer). Record the results of these tests using accepted forms and procedures.

3. Using surface anatomy, palpate or draw the origins and course of each ligament in list C.

4. Using surface anatomy, palpate the origin, insertion, and course of each muscle in list D. Also, tell the major function of each muscle.

5. Using surface anatomy, palpate each structure in list E.

Injury Assessment

6. Obtain the medical history of an athlete with a suspected arm or elbow injury.

7. Demonstrate proper administration and interpretation of the special tests in list F.

8. Demonstrate how you would observe and identify the clinical signs and symptoms associated with the injuries and conditions in list G.

9. Explain and demonstrate the mechanisms by which each injury in list G occurs. Name the three sports in which each injury is most likely to occur and explain any differences among the injury occurrences and mechanisms in those sports.

10. Demonstrate appropriate sensory, circulatory, and neurological tests for the injuries in list G.

11. Palpate and assess the integrity of the bones and soft tissues associated with each injury in list G.

12. Perform special tests to assess the integrity of the joints involved in each injury in list G and explain how you would interpret these tests.

13. Demonstrate the use of manual muscle testing and other tests as appropriate to assess the flexibility and strength of the muscles associated with each injury in list G.

14. Demonstrate functional and activity-specific tests to determine the integrity of each structure involved in each injury in list G.

Proficiency Demonstration

1. Develop appropriate subject knowledge through coursework (C), verbal conversation (V), quizzes (Q), worksheets (W), or other approved activities (O).

2. Practice and reinforce the skills in clinical skills and laboratory courses.

3. Refine your skills by observing peer teachers and clinical instructors as they perform the skills (preferably on patients), discussing the competencies with peer teachers and clinical instructors, practicing alone and with others, and then demonstrating proficiency to a peer teacher.

4. Demonstrate your proficiency to an ACI.

APPROVED BY
(date and signature, and mode for didactic)

1. Bones
   Didactic _____
   Lab _____
   Peer _____
   ACI _____

2. Articulations
   Didactic _____
   Lab _____
   Peer _____
   ACI _____

3. Ligaments
   Didactic _____
   Lab _____
   Peer _____
   ACI _____

4. Muscles

Didactic _____

Lab _____

Peer _____

ACI _____

5. Other structures

Didactic _____

Lab _____

Peer _____

ACI _____

6. History

Didactic _____

Lab _____

Peer _____

ACI _____

7. Special tests

Symmetry, carrying angle (cubital valgus and varus), efficiency of movement

Didactic _____

Lab _____

Peer _____

ACI _____

Valgus stress test

Didactic _____

Lab _____

Peer _____

ACI _____

Varus stress test

Didactic _____

Lab _____

Peer _____

ACI _____

Moving valgus stress test

Didactic _____

Lab _____

Peer _____

ACI _____

Cozen's (tennis elbow) test

Didactic _____

Lab _____

Peer _____

ACI _____

Resistive tennis elbow test

Didactic _____

Lab _____

Peer _____

ACI _____

Passive tennis elbow test

Didactic _____

Lab _____

Peer _____

ACI _____

Medial epicondylitis (golfer's elbow) test

Didactic _____

Lab _____

Peer _____

ACI _____

Hyperextension test

Didactic _____

Lab _____

Peer _____

ACI _____

Tinel's sign

Didactic _____

Lab _____

Peer _____

ACI _____

8-14. Complete competencies 8 through 14 for the injuries or conditions in list G:

Bicipital strain

Didactic _____

Lab _____

Peer _____

ACI _____

Humeral fracture

Didactic _____

Lab _____

Peer _____

ACI _____

Epiphyseal fracture

Didactic _____

Lab _____

Peer _____

ACI _____

Humeral contusion

Didactic _____

Lab _____

Peer _____

ACI _____

Humeral exostoses

Didactic _____

Lab _____

Peer _____

ACI _____

Supracondylar fracture

Didactic _____

Lab _____

Peer _____

ACI _____

Olecranon bursitis

Didactic _____

Lab _____

Peer _____

ACI _____

Medial elbow strain

Didactic _____

Lab _____

Peer _____

ACI _____

Medial collateral ligament sprain

Didactic _____

Lab _____

Peer _____

ACI _____

Elbow hyperextension

Didactic _____

Lab _____

Peer _____

ACI _____

Elbow dislocation

Didactic _____

Lab _____

Peer _____

ACI _____

Elbow fracture

Didactic _____

Lab _____

Peer _____

ACI _____

Radial nerve injury

Didactic _____

Lab _____

Peer _____

ACI _____

Throwing injury

Didactic _____

Lab _____

Peer _____

ACI _____

Medial epicondylitis

Didactic _____

Lab _____

Peer _____

ACI _____

Lateral epicondylitis

Didactic _____

Lab _____

Peer _____

ACI _____

Forearm contusion

Didactic _____

Lab _____

Peer _____

ACI _____

Radial head fracture

Didactic _____

Lab _____

Peer _____

ACI _____

Forearm splint

Didactic _____

Lab _____

Peer _____

ACI _____

Dislocation or subluxation

Didactic _____

Lab _____

Peer _____

ACI _____

Pronator teres syndrome

Didactic _____

Lab _____

Peer _____

ACI _____

Nerve injury

Didactic _____

Lab _____

Peer _____

ACI _____

Bursitis

Didactic _____

Lab _____

Peer _____

ACI _____

Osteochondritis dissecans

Didactic _____

Lab _____

Peer _____

ACI _____

COMMENTS

_____

_____

_____

_____

_____

_____

Wrist and Hand Injury Assessment and Diagnosis

Objective

Develop and demonstrate the skills necessary to evaluate wrist and hand injuries.

NATA Athletic Training Educational Competencies embedded in this module: AC-C6, DI-C6, DI-C7, DI-C10, DI-C12, DI-C13, DI-C15, DI-C16, DI-C17, DI-P1, DI-P2, DI-P4, DI-P5, DI-P6, DI-P7, DI-P8, DI-P10, DI-CP1

Anatomy and Conditions for This Module

A. Bones and Prominent Bony Features

- Ulna
  - Styloid process
  - Head
  - Distal radioulnar joint
- Radius
  - Styloid process
  - Distal radioulnar joint
- Pisiform
- Triquetrum
- Lunate
- Scaphoid
- Hamate
- Capitate
- Trapezoid
- Trapezium
- Metacarpals
- Phalanges
  - Proximal
  - Middle
  - Distal

B. Articulations

- Distal radioulnar
- Radiocarpal
- Ulnocarpal
- Midcarpal
- Carpal-metacarpal
- Proximal interphalangeal
- Distal interphalangeal

C. Ligaments

- Flexor retinaculum
- Ulnar collateral
- Radial collateral
- PIP
- DIP
- Palmar
- Deep transverse
- Volar plate

D. Muscles

- Palmaris longus
- Extensor pollicis longus
- Flexor carpi radialis
- Flexor carpi ulnaris
- Brachioradialis
- Extensor carpi radialis
- Extensor carpi ulnaris
- Extensor digitorum
- Lumbricles
- Palmer interossei
- Dorsal interossei

E. Other Structures

- Medial nerve
- Radial nerve
- Ulnar nerve
- Radial pulse
- Thenar eminence
- Hypothenar eminence

F. Special Tests

- Finkelstein's test
- Valgus stress test
- Varus stress test
- Glide test
- Triangular Fibro Cartilage Complex (TFCC) compression test
- Tinel's sign
- Phalen's test
- Tap or percussion test
- Long bone compression test
- Watson test
- Murphy's sign

G. Injuries and Conditions

- Colles' fracture
- Scaphoid fracture
- Lunate dislocation

- Hamate fracture
- Bennett's fracture
- Carpal (boxer's) fracture
- Radioulnar sprain
- Wrist ganglion
- Carpal sprain
- Carpal tunnel syndrome
- Hand contusion
- Dupuytren's contracture
- Ganglion
- Bishop's or benediction deformity
- Ape hand
- Claw fingers
- Drop-wrist deformity
- Volkmann's contracture
- Metacarpal fracture
- Phalangeal fracture
- Thumb ulnocollateral ligament sprain
- PIP sprain
- Flexor tendon avulsion (jersey finger)
- Extensor tendon avulsion (mallet finger)
- Extensor tendon rupture (boutonniere deformity)
- Volar plate rupture (pseudoboutonniere deformity)
- Interphalangeal dislocations
- Subungual hematoma
- Clubbed nails
- Spoon-shaped nails
- Swan neck deformity
- Trigger finger

Competencies

Note: All procedures must be performed.

Anatomical Review and Assessment of Structural Integrity

1. Name and palpate each bone and bony structure in list A. Tell what differences you would expect to feel if the bone were fractured.

2. Palpate or draw the joint line for each articulation in list B. Then perform active and passive joint ROM tests using both qualitative and quantitative techniques (e.g., tape measure, goniometer, and inclinometer). Record the results of these tests using accepted forms and procedures.

3. Using surface anatomy, palpate or draw the origins and course of each ligament in list C.

4. Using surface anatomy, palpate the origin, insertion, and course of each muscle in list D. Also, tell the major function of each muscle.

5. Using surface anatomy, palpate each structure in list E.

Injury Assessment

6. Obtain the medical history of an athlete with a suspected wrist or hand injury.

7. Demonstrate proper administration and interpretation of the special tests in list F.

8. Demonstrate how you would observe and identify the clinical signs and symptoms associated with the injuries and conditions in list G.

9. Explain and demonstrate the mechanisms by which each injury in list G occurs. Name the three sports in which each injury is most likely to occur and explain any differences among the injury occurrences and mechanisms in those sports.

10. Demonstrate appropriate sensory, circulatory, and neurological tests for the injuries in list G.

11. Palpate and assess the integrity of the bones and soft tissues associated with each injury in list G.

12. Perform special tests to assess the integrity of the joints involved in each injury in list G and explain how you would interpret these tests.

13. Demonstrate the use of manual muscle testing and other tests as appropriate to assess the flexibility and strength of the muscles associated with each injury in list G.

14. Demonstrate functional and activity-specific tests to determine the integrity of each structure involved in each injury in list G.

Proficiency Demonstration

1. Develop appropriate subject knowledge through coursework (C), verbal conversation (V), quizzes (Q), worksheets (W), or other approved activities (O).

2. Practice and reinforce the skills in clinical skills and laboratory courses.

3. Refine your skills by observing peer teachers and clinical instructors as they perform the skills (preferably on patients), discussing the competencies with peer teachers and clinical instructors, practicing alone and with others, and then demonstrating proficiency to a peer teacher.

4. Demonstrate your proficiency to an ACI.

APPROVED BY
(date and signature, and mode for didactic)

1. Bones
   Didactic _____
   Lab _____
   Peer _____
   ACI _____

2. Articulations
   Didactic _____
   Lab _____
   Peer _____
   ACI _____

3. Ligaments
   Didactic _____
   Lab _____
   Peer _____
   ACI _____

4. Muscles
   Didactic _____
   Lab _____
   Peer _____
   ACI _____

5. Other structures
   Didactic _____
   Lab _____
   Peer _____
   ACI _____

6. History
   Didactic _____
   Lab _____
   Peer _____
   ACI _____

7. Special tests
   Finkelstein's test
   Didactic _____
   Lab _____
   Peer _____
   ACI _____

Valgus stress test
Didactic _____
Lab _____
Peer _____
ACI _____

Varus stress test
Didactic _____
Lab _____
Peer _____
ACI _____

Glide test
Didactic _____
Lab _____
Peer _____
ACI _____

TFCC compression test
Didactic _____
Lab _____
Peer _____
ACI _____

Tinel's sign
Didactic _____
Lab _____
Peer _____
ACI _____

Phalen's test
Didactic _____
Lab _____
Peer _____
ACI _____

Tap or percussion test
Didactic _____
Lab _____
Peer _____
ACI _____

Long bone compression test

Didactic _____

Lab _____

Peer _____

ACI _____

Watson test

Didactic _____

Lab _____

Peer _____

ACI _____

Murphy's sign

Didactic _____

Lab _____

Peer _____

ACI _____

8-14. Complete competencies 8 through 14 for the injuries or conditions in list G:

Colles' fracture

Didactic _____

Lab _____

Peer _____

ACI _____

Scaphoid fracture

Didactic _____

Lab _____

Peer _____

ACI _____

Lunate dislocation

Didactic _____

Lab _____

Peer _____

ACI _____

Hamate fracture

Didactic _____

Lab _____

Peer _____

ACI _____

Bennett's fracture

Didactic _____

Lab _____

Peer _____

ACI _____

Carpal (boxer's) fracture

Didactic _____

Lab _____

Peer _____

ACI _____

Radioulnar sprain

Didactic _____

Lab _____

Peer _____

ACI _____

Wrist ganglion

Didactic _____

Lab _____

Peer _____

ACI _____

Carpal sprain

Didactic _____

Lab _____

Peer _____

ACI _____

Carpal tunnel syndrome

Didactic _____

Lab _____

Peer _____

ACI _____

Hand contusion

Didactic _____

Lab _____

Peer _____

ACI _____

Dupuytren's contracture

Didactic _____

Lab _____

Peer _____

ACI _____

Ganglion

Didactic _____

Lab _____

Peer _____

ACI _____

Bishop's or benediction deformity

Didactic _____

Lab _____

Peer _____

ACI _____

Ape hand

Didactic _____

Lab _____

Peer _____

ACI _____

Claw fingers

Didactic _____

Lab _____

Peer _____

ACI _____

Drop-wrist deformity

Didactic _____

Lab _____

Peer _____

ACI _____

Volkmann's contracture

Didactic _____

Lab _____

Peer _____

ACI _____

Metacarpal fracture

Didactic _____

Lab _____

Peer _____

ACI _____

Phalangeal fracture

Didactic _____

Lab _____

Peer _____

ACI _____

Thumb ulnocollateral ligament sprain

Didactic _____

Lab _____

Peer _____

ACI _____

PIP sprain

Didactic _____

Lab _____

Peer _____

ACI _____

Flexor tendon avulsion

Didactic _____

Lab _____

Peer _____

ACI _____

Extensor tendon avulsion

Didactic _____

Lab _____

Peer _____

ACI _____

Extensor tendon rupture

Didactic _____

Lab _____

Peer _____

ACI _____

Volar plate rupture

Didactic _____

Lab _____

Peer _____

ACI _____

Interphalangeal dislocations

Didactic _____

Lab _____

Peer _____

ACI _____

Subungual hematoma

Didactic _____

Lab _____

Peer _____

ACI _____

Clubbed nails

Didactic _____

Lab _____

Peer _____

ACI _____

Spoon-shaped nails

Didactic _____

Lab _____

Peer _____

ACI _____

Swan neck deformity

Didactic _____

Lab _____

Peer _____

ACI _____

Trigger finger

Didactic _____

Lab _____

Peer _____

ACI _____

COMMENTS

_____

_____

_____

_____

_____

_____

_____

Cervical Spine Injury Assessment and Diagnosis

Objective

Develop and demonstrate the skills necessary to evaluate cervical spine injuries.

NATA Athletic Training Educational Competencies embedded in this module: AC-C6, AC-C22, DI-C6, DI-C7, DI-C8, DI-C9, DI-C10, DI-C11, DI-C12, DI-C13, DI-C15, DI-C16, DI-C17, DI-P1, DI-P2, DI-P3, DI-P4, DI-P5, DI-P6, DI-P7, DI-P8, DI-P9, DI-P10, DI-CP1

Anatomy and Conditions for This Module

A. Bones and Prominent Bony Features

- Cervical vertebrae
  - Spinous processes
  - Transverse processes
- Atlas
- Axis
- Clavicle
- First rib

B. Articulations

- Cervical intervertebral articulation
- Alanto-occipital articulation
- Alanto-axial articulation

C. Ligaments

- Nuchal
- Ligamentum flavum
- Ligamentum nuchae

D. Muscles

- Sternocleidomastoid
- Scalene (three portions)
- Trapezius
- Posterior vertebral

E. Other Structures

- Brachial plexus
- Myotomes
- Dermatomes
- Cervical plexus
- Vertebral artery

F. Special Tests

- Valsalva maneuver
- Foraminal distraction and compression test
- Spurling's test
- Shoulder depression (brachial plexus tension) test
- Vertebral artery test
- Tinel's sign
- Upper-extremity neurological examination (upper-quarter screen)

G. Injuries and Conditions

- Cervical dislocation
- Cervical subluxation
- Cervical sprain
- Cervical strain
- Neck contusion
- Neck burner
- Neck muscle atrophy
- Vertebral fracture
- Faulty head and neck posture
- Intervertebral disc herniation
- Nerve root compression or stretch
- Spinal cord ischemia
- Torticollis
- Brachial plexus neuropathy
- Neurovascular dysfunction
- Vertebral artery occlusion

Competencies

Note: All procedures must be performed.

Anatomical Review and Assessment of Structural Integrity

1. Name and palpate each bone and bony structure in list A. Tell what differences you would expect to feel if the bone were fractured.

2. Palpate or draw the joint line for each articulation in list B. Then perform active and passive joint ROM tests using both qualitative and quantitative techniques (e.g., tape measure, goniometer, and inclinometer). Record the results of these tests using accepted forms and procedures.

3. Using surface anatomy, palpate or draw the origins and course of each ligament in list C.

4. Using surface anatomy, palpate the origin, insertion, and course of each muscle in list D. Also, tell the major function of each muscle.

5. Using surface anatomy, palpate each structure in list E.

Injury Assessment

6. Obtain the medical history of an athlete with a suspected cervical spine injury.

7. Demonstrate proper administration and interpretation of the special tests in list F.

8. Demonstrate how you would observe and identify the clinical signs and symptoms associated with the injuries and conditions in list G.

9. Explain and demonstrate the mechanisms by which each injury in list G occurs. Name the three sports in which each injury is most likely to occur and explain any differences among the injury occurrences and mechanisms in those sports.

10. Demonstrate appropriate sensory, circulatory, and neurological tests for the injuries in list G.

11. Palpate and assess the integrity of the bones and soft tissues associated with each injury in list G.

12. Perform special tests to assess the integrity of the joints involved in each injury in list G and explain how you would interpret these tests.

13. Demonstrate the use of manual muscle testing and other tests as appropriate to assess the flexibility and strength of the muscles associated with each injury in list G.

14. Demonstrate functional and activity-specific tests to determine the integrity of each structure involved in each injury in list G.

Proficiency Demonstration

1. Develop appropriate subject knowledge through coursework (C), verbal conversation (V), quizzes (Q), worksheets (W), or other approved activities (O).

2. Practice and reinforce the skills in clinical skills and laboratory courses.

3. Refine your skills by observing peer teachers and clinical instructors as they perform the skills (preferably on patients), discussing the competencies with peer teachers and clinical instructors, practicing alone and with others, and then demonstrating proficiency to a peer teacher.

4. Demonstrate your proficiency to an ACI.

APPROVED BY
(date and signature, and mode for didactic)

1. Bones

   Didactic _____

   Lab _____

   Peer _____

   ACI _____

2. Articulations

   Didactic _____

   Lab _____

   Peer _____

   ACI _____

3. Ligaments

   Didactic _____

   Lab _____

   Peer _____

   ACI _____

4. Muscles

   Didactic _____

   Lab _____

   Peer _____

   ACI _____

5. Other structures

   Didactic _____

   Lab _____

   Peer _____

   ACI _____

6. History

   Didactic _____

   Lab _____

   Peer _____

   ACI _____

7. Special tests

   Valsalva maneuver

   Didactic _____

   Lab _____

   Peer _____

   ACI _____

LEVEL
2.9

MODULE
J11

Foraminal distraction and compression test

Didactic _____

Lab _____

Peer _____

ACI _____

Spurling's test

Didactic _____

Lab _____

Peer _____

ACI _____

Shoulder depression (brachial plexus tension) test

Didactic _____

Lab _____

Peer _____

ACI _____

Vertebral artery test

Didactic _____

Lab _____

Peer _____

ACI _____

Tinel's sign

Didactic _____

Lab _____

Peer _____

ACI _____

Upper-extremity neurological examination (upper-quarter screen)

Didactic _____

Lab _____

Peer _____

ACI _____

8-14. Complete competencies 8 through 14 for the injuries or conditions in list G:

Cervical dislocation

Didactic _____

Lab _____

Peer _____

ACI _____

Cervical subluxation

Didactic _____

Lab _____

Peer _____

ACI _____

Cervical sprain

Didactic _____

Lab _____

Peer _____

ACI _____

Cervical strain

Didactic _____

Lab _____

Peer _____

ACI _____

Neck contusion

Didactic _____

Lab _____

Peer _____

ACI _____

Neck burner

Didactic _____

Lab _____

Peer _____

ACI _____

Neck muscle atrophy

Didactic _____

Lab _____

Peer _____

ACI _____

Vertebral fracture

Didactic _____

Lab _____

Peer _____

ACI _____

Faulty head and neck posture

Didactic _____

Lab _____

Peer _____

ACI _____

Intervertebral disc herniation

Didactic _____

Lab _____

Peer _____

ACI _____

Nerve root compression or stretch

Didactic _____

Lab _____

Peer _____

ACI _____

Spinal cord ischemia

Didactic _____

Lab _____

Peer _____

ACI _____

Torticollis

Didactic _____

Lab _____

Peer _____

ACI _____

Brachial plexus neuropathy

Didactic _____

Lab _____

Peer _____

ACI _____

Neurovascular dysfunction

Didactic _____

Lab _____

Peer _____

ACI _____

Vertebral artery occlusion

Didactic _____

Lab _____

Peer _____

ACI _____

COMMENTS

_____

_____

_____

_____

_____

Head and Facial Injury Assessment and Diagnosis

Objective

Develop and demonstrate the skills necessary to evaluate head and facial injuries.

NATA Athletic Training Educational Competencies embedded in this module: DI-C6, DI-C7, DI-C8, DI-C9, DI-C10, DI-C13, DI-C16, DI-C17, DI-P1, DI-P2, DI-P4, DI-P8, DI-P9, DI-P10, DI-CP1, AC-C2, AC-C22, AC-P4, MC-C3, MC-C4, MC-C5, MC-C6, MC-C21, MC-P1, MC-P2

Anatomy and Conditions for This Module

A. Bones and Prominent Bony Features

- Skull
  - Parietal
  - Occipital
  - Frontal
  - Temporal
- Mastoid process
- Mandible
- Maxilla
- Nasal (both)
- Zygomatic arch
- Ethmoid
- Sphenoid
- Teeth

B. Articulations (Temporomandibular Joint [TMJ])

C. Other Structures

- Nasal passages
- Auris
  - Aurice (pinna)
  - External auditory canal
  - Tympanic membrane
  - Ossicles
  - Cochlea
  - Semicircular canals
- Eye
  - Cornea
  - Lens
  - Iris
  - Anterior chamber
  - Posterior chamber
  - Conjunctiva
  - Retina

D. Special Tests

- Level of consciousness
- Amnesia (retrograde or posttraumatic)
- Orientation (person, time, place orientation)
- Balance and coordination tests (e.g., BESS, Rhomberg, tandem walking, finger to nose)
- Pulse, blood pressure
- Cranial nerves (e.g., eye motion, facial muscles)
- Cognitive tests (e.g., recall, serial sevens, digit span)
- Spinal nerve roots (e.g., upper-quarter screen)
- TMJ palpation test
- Bite (tongue blade) test
- Battle's sign
- Raccoon eye sign

E. Injuries and Conditions

- Head and face
  - Skull fracture
  - Jaw fracture
  - Scalp hematoma
  - Facial laceration
  - Concussion
  - Intracranial bleeding
  - Headache
- Eye
  - Foreign body in the eye
  - Contact lens lost in the eye
  - Lens or iris injury
  - Orbital blowout fracture
  - Conjunctivitis (pink eye)
  - Corneal abrasion
  - Corneal laceration
  - Detached retina
  - Hyphema (eye chamber hemorrhage)
  - Stye
- Ear
  - Impacted cerumen
  - Otitis externa (swimmer's ear)
  - Otitis media
  - Hematoma auris (cauliflower ear)
  - Ruptured eardrum
  - Foreign body in the ear
- Nose
  - Deviated septum
  - Epistaxis (nose bleed)
  - Nasal fracture

- Jaw, mouth, and teeth
  - Gingivitis
  - Mandibular fracture
  - Maxilla fracture
  - Periodontitis
  - TMJ dislocation
  - TMJ dysfunction
  - Tooth abscess
  - Tooth extrusion
  - Tooth fracture
  - Tooth intrusion
  - Tooth luxation

Competencies

Note: All procedures must be performed.

Anatomical Review and Assessment of Structural Integrity

1. Name and palpate each bone and bony structure in list A. Tell what differences you would expect to feel if the bone were fractured.

2. Palpate the TMJ. Then perform active and passive joint ROM tests using both qualitative and quantitative techniques (e.g., tape measure, goniometer, and inclinometer). Record the results of these tests using accepted forms and procedures.

3. Identify, and palpate as possible, each structure in list C.

Injury Assessment

4. Obtain the medical history of an athlete with a suspected head injury.

5. Demonstrate proper administration and interpretation of the special tests in list D.

6. Demonstrate how you would observe and identify the clinical signs and symptoms associated with the injuries and conditions in list E.

7. Explain and demonstrate the mechanisms by which each injury in list E occurs. Name the three sports in which each injury is most likely to occur and explain any differences among the injury occurrences and mechanisms in those sports.

8. Demonstrate appropriate sensory, circulatory, and neurological tests for the injuries in list E.

9. Palpate and assess the integrity of the bones and soft tissues associated with each injury in list E.

10. Demonstrate functional and activity-specific tests to determine the integrity of each structure involved in each injury in list E.

Injury Assessment and Diagnosis

11. Explain and demonstrate the appropriate immediate care procedures for each injury in list E. Explain the objectives and criteria for progressing from each step to the next in the procedure.

12. Demonstrate a complete rehabilitation program for each injury in list E. As you proceed, explain the objectives and procedures of each step in the program. Explain the measurement criteria for advancing from one step to another.

Proficiency Demonstration

1. Develop appropriate subject knowledge through coursework (C), verbal conversation (V), quizzes (Q), worksheets (W), or other approved activities (O).

2. Practice and reinforce the skills in clinical skills and laboratory courses.

3. Refine your skills by observing peer teachers and clinical instructors as they perform the skills (preferably on patients), discussing the competencies with peer teachers and clinical instructors, practicing alone and with others, and then demonstrating proficiency to a peer teacher.

4. Demonstrate your proficiency to an ACI.

APPROVED BY
(date and signature, and mode for didactic)

1. Bones

   Didactic _____

   Lab _____

   Peer _____

   ACI _____

2. Articulations

   Didactic _____

   Lab _____

   Peer _____

   ACI _____

3. Other structures

   Didactic _____

   Lab _____

   Peer _____

   ACI _____

LEVEL
2.9

MODULE
J12

4. History

Didactic _____

Lab _____

Peer _____

ACI _____

5. Special tests

Level of consciousness

Didactic _____

Lab _____

Peer _____

ACI _____

Amnesia (retrograde or posttraumatic)

Didactic _____

Lab _____

Peer _____

ACI _____

Levels of consciousness

Didactic _____

Lab _____

Peer _____

ACI _____

Orientation (person, time, place orientation)

Didactic _____

Lab _____

Peer _____

ACI _____

Balance and coordination tests (e.g., BESS, Rhomberg, tandem walking, finger to nose)

Didactic _____

Lab _____

Peer _____

ACI _____

Pulse, blood pressure

Didactic _____

Lab _____

Peer _____

ACI _____

Cranial nerves (e.g., eye motion, facial muscles)

Didactic _____

Lab _____

Peer _____

ACI _____

Cognitive tests (e.g., recall, serial sevens, digit span)

Didactic _____

Lab _____

Peer _____

ACI _____

Spinal nerve roots (e.g., upper-quarter screen)

Didactic _____

Lab _____

Peer _____

ACI _____

TMJ palpation test

Didactic _____

Lab _____

Peer _____

ACI _____

Bite (tongue blade) test

Didactic _____

Lab _____

Peer _____

ACI _____

Battle's sign

Didactic _____

Lab _____

Peer _____

ACI _____

Raccoon eye sign

Didactic _____

Lab _____

Peer _____

ACI _____

6-12. Complete competencies 6 through 12 for the injuries or conditions in list E:

Head and face

– Skull fracture

Didactic _____

Lab _____

Peer _____

ACI _____

– Jaw fracture

Didactic _____

Lab _____

Peer _____

ACI _____

– Scalp hematoma

Didactic _____

Lab _____

Peer _____

ACI _____

– Facial laceration

Didactic _____

Lab _____

Peer _____

ACI _____

– Concussion

Didactic _____

Lab _____

Peer _____

ACI _____

– Intracranial bleeding

Didactic _____

Lab _____

Peer _____

ACI _____

– Headache

Didactic _____

Lab _____

Peer _____

ACI _____

Eye

– Foreign body in the eye

Didactic _____

Lab _____

Peer _____

ACI _____

– Contact lens lost in the eye

Didactic _____

Lab _____

Peer _____

ACI _____

– Lens or iris injury

Didactic _____

Lab _____

Peer _____

ACI _____

– Orbital blowout fracture

Didactic _____

Lab _____

Peer _____

ACI _____

– Conjunctivitis

Didactic _____

Lab _____

Peer _____

ACI _____

– Corneal abrasion

Didactic _____

Lab _____

Peer _____

ACI _____

– Corneal laceration

Didactic _____

Lab _____

Peer _____

ACI _____

– Detached retina

Didactic _____

Lab _____

Peer _____

ACI _____

– Hyphema

Didactic _____

Lab _____

Peer _____

ACI _____

– Stye

Didactic _____

Lab _____

Peer _____

ACI _____

Ear

– Impacted cerumen

Didactic _____

Lab _____

Peer _____

ACI _____

– Otitis externa

Didactic _____

Lab _____

Peer _____

ACI _____

– Otitis media

Didactic _____

Lab _____

Peer _____

ACI _____

– Hematoma auris

Didactic _____

Lab _____

Peer _____

ACI _____

– Ruptured eardrum

Didactic _____

Lab _____

Peer _____

ACI _____

– Foreign body in the ear

Didactic _____

Lab _____

Peer _____

ACI _____

Nose

– Deviated septum

Didactic _____

Lab _____

Peer _____

ACI _____

– Epistaxis

Didactic _____

Lab _____

Peer _____

ACI _____

– Nasal fracture

Didactic _____

Lab _____

Peer _____

ACI _____

Jaw, mouth, and teeth

– Gingivitis

Didactic _____

Lab _____

Peer _____

ACI _____

– Mandibular fracture

Didactic _____

Lab _____

Peer _____

ACI _____

– Maxilla fracture

Didactic _____

Lab _____

Peer _____

ACI _____

– Periodontitis

Didactic _____

Lab _____

Peer _____

ACI _____

– TMJ dislocation

Didactic _____

Lab _____

Peer _____

ACI _____

– TMJ dysfunction

Didactic _____

Lab _____

Peer _____

ACI _____

– Tooth abscess

Didactic _____

Lab _____

Peer _____

ACI _____

– Tooth extrusion

Didactic _____

Lab _____

Peer _____

ACI _____

– Tooth fracture

Didactic _____

Lab _____

Peer _____

ACI _____

– Tooth intrusion

Didactic _____

Lab _____

Peer _____

ACI _____

– Tooth luxation

Didactic _____

Lab _____

Peer _____

ACI _____

COMMENTS

_____

_____

_____

_____

_____

_____

_____

Level 2.10

General Medical Conditions, Disorders, and Diseases

In many employment settings the AT is the primary resource for all medical concerns. ATs manage orthopedic and sport performance issues relating to the muscular and skeletal systems, as well as medical conditions involving the cardiovascular, digestive, endocrine, excretory, immune, integumentary, nervous, reproductive, and respiratory systems. ATs have developed a reputation for being knowledgeable health care practitioners and therefore are often asked questions regarding multiple conditions, diseases, and disabilities. Being able to recognize pathology that needs referral and treatment is critical to management of medical conditions.

Appropriate recognition, referral, and treatment may not only save time loss from competition, but in some cases it may save a life. ATs must become competent in managing injury, illness, and disease that affect the head, brain, face, eyes, ears, nose, throat, skin, heart, lungs, abdominal organs, and body systems.

In order to adequately answer questions about and manage the care for general medical anomalies, the AT must have a working knowledge of the normal function and response to exercise of the body systems and organs. Much of the knowledge regarding function and response to exercise will be covered in didactic classes. It is important to understand this basic knowledge and become familiar with normal functions and abilities of the systems and organs. This knowledge along with the clinical skills necessary to perform assessment, evaluation, and screening procedures will help determine when an underlying pathology might exist.

Discussions and classroom work explaining referral and treatment options must also be completed so that ATs can appropriately manage the medical conditions of their patients. As with orthopedic injuries, appropriate assessment and referral of general medical conditions is essential to proper management and in some cases might be critical to a full recovery.

Over the course of the modules in this section, the student will be asked to describe the normal function of many organ systems, organs, and other structures. The student will also be asked to perform assessment and screening procedures to determine if a referral to another allied health professional is needed. Basic knowledge of function, detection of abnormalities, referral procedures, and treatment options for non-orthopedic medical conditions should be evaluated using various methods, including quizzes, tests, O/P evaluations, and simulations.

Assessment, Diagnosis, and Care
of Simple Dermatological Conditions

Objective

Develop and demonstrate the skills necessary to evaluate, care for, and prevent simple dermatological conditions.

NATA Athletic Training Educational Competencies embedded in this module: AC-C30, AC-P4, MC-C15, MC-C16, MC-C19

Conditions for This Module

- Abscess
- Acne vulgaris
- Blister
- Carbuncle
- Cellulitis
- Molluscum contagiosum
- Dermatitis
- Eczema
- Folliculitis
- Frostbite
- Furunculosis
- Herpes simplex
- Tinea versicolor
- Pediculosis
- Herpes zoster
- Hives
- Impetigo
- Psoriasis
- Ringworm
- Scabies
- Sebaceous cyst
- Tinea cruris
- Tinea pedis
- Urticaria
- Verruca plantaris
- Verruca vulgaris
- Tinea capitis

Competencies

1. Describe, with the use of pictures, the structure of the skin (including all the layers).

2. Describe, with the use of pictures if necessary, the signs, symptoms, and predisposing conditions associated with the diseases and conditions listed in this module. If any conditions are more prevalent in specific sports, identify those sports.

3. Explain and demonstrate the appropriate assessment and diagnosis procedures for each condition.

4. Explain and demonstrate, if possible, the appropriate management of each condition.

5. Explain the impact of each condition on sport participation.

Proficiency Demonstration

1. Develop appropriate subject knowledge through coursework (C), verbal conversation (V), quizzes (Q), worksheets (W), or other approved activities (O).

2. Practice and reinforce the skills in clinical skills and laboratory courses.

3. Refine your skills by observing peer teachers and clinical instructors as they perform the skills (preferably on patients), discussing the competencies with peer teachers and clinical instructors, practicing alone and with others, and then demonstrating proficiency to a peer teacher.

4. Demonstrate your proficiency to an ACI.

APPROVED BY
(date and signature, and mode for didactic)

1. Skin structure

Didactic _____

Lab _____

Peer _____

ACI _____

2-5. Complete competencies 2 through 5 for the following conditions:

Abscess

Didactic _____

Lab _____

Peer _____

ACI _____

Acne vulgaris

Didactic _____

Lab _____

Peer _____

ACI _____

Blister

Didactic _____

Lab _____

Peer _____

ACI _____

Carbuncle

Didactic _____

Lab _____

Peer _____

ACI _____

Cellulitis

Didactic _____

Lab _____

Peer _____

ACI _____

Molluscum contagiosum

Didactic _____

Lab _____

Peer _____

ACI _____

Dermatitis

Didactic _____

Lab _____

Peer _____

ACI _____

Eczema

Didactic _____

Lab _____

Peer _____

ACI _____

Folliculitis

Didactic _____

Lab _____

Peer _____

ACI _____

Frostbite

Didactic _____

Lab _____

Peer _____

ACI _____

Furunculosis

Didactic _____

Lab _____

Peer _____

ACI _____

Herpes simplex

Didactic _____

Lab _____

Peer _____

ACI _____

Tinea versicolor

Didactic _____

Lab _____

Peer _____

ACI _____

Pediculosis

Didactic _____

Lab _____

Peer _____

ACI _____

Herpes zoster

Didactic _____

Lab _____

Peer _____

ACI _____

Hives

Didactic _____

Lab _____

Peer _____

ACI _____

Impetigo

Didactic _____

Lab _____

Peer _____

ACI _____

Psoriasis

Didactic _____

Lab _____

Peer _____

ACI _____

Ringworm

Didactic _____

Lab _____

Peer _____

ACI _____

Scabies

Didactic _____

Lab _____

Peer _____

ACI _____

Sebaceous cysts

Didactic _____

Lab _____

Peer _____

ACI _____

Tinea cruris

Didactic _____

Lab _____

Peer _____

ACI _____

Tinea pedis

Didactic _____

Lab _____

Peer _____

ACI _____

Urticaria

Didactic _____

Lab _____

Peer _____

ACI _____

Verruca plantaris

Didactic _____

Lab _____

Peer _____

ACI _____

Verruca vulgaris

Didactic _____

Lab _____

Peer _____

ACI _____

Tinea capitis

Didactic _____

Lab _____

Peer _____

ACI _____

COMMENTS

_____

_____

_____

_____

_____

Common Syndromes and Diseases

Objective

Develop and demonstrate the skills necessary to evaluate, care for, and prevent common syndromes and diseases.

NATA Athletic Training Educational Competencies embedded in this module: AC-P4, MC-C1, MC-C2, MC-C3, MC-C13, MC-C16, MC-C19, MC-C20, MC-P4, RM-C15

Syndromes and Diseases for This Module

- Diabetes
- Hyperthyroidism
- Hypothyroidism
- Pancreatitis
- Infectious mononucleosis
- Measles
- Mumps
- Epilepsy
- Syncope
- Reflex sympathetic dystrophy
- Meningitis
- Iron-deficiency anemia (systemic)
- Sickle cell anemia (systemic)
- Lyme disease

Competencies

1. Describe, with the use of pictures if necessary, the signs, symptoms, and predisposing conditions associated with the following syndromes and diseases. Tell how each condition affects athletes' performances in American football, basketball, baseball and softball, track and field, and two other sports.

2. Explain, and demonstrate if possible, the appropriate management procedures for each condition listed in this module. Explain the objectives and criteria for progressing for each step in the procedure.

3. Explain guidelines for participation (practice and games) for athletes with each condition.

4. Demonstrate or explain procedures for preventing each condition.

Proficiency Demonstration

1. Develop appropriate subject knowledge through coursework (C), verbal conversation (V), quizzes (Q), worksheets (W), or other approved activities (O).

2. Practice and reinforce the skills in clinical skills and laboratory courses.

3. Refine your skills by observing peer teachers and clinical instructors as they perform the skills (preferably on patients), discussing the competencies with peer teachers and clinical instructors, practicing alone and with others, and then demonstrating proficiency to a peer teacher.

4. Demonstrate your proficiency to an ACI.

APPROVED BY
(date and signature, and mode for didactic)

1-4. Complete competencies 1 through 4 for the following symptoms or diseases:

Diabetes

Didactic _____

Lab _____

Peer _____

ACI _____

Hyperthyroidism

Didactic _____

Lab _____

Peer _____

ACI _____

Hypothyroidism

Didactic _____

Lab _____

Peer _____

ACI _____

Pancreatitis

Didactic _____

Lab _____

Peer _____

ACI _____

Infectious mononucleosis

Didactic _____

Lab _____

Peer _____

ACI _____

Measles

Didactic _____

Lab _____

Peer _____

ACI _____

Mumps

Didactic _____

Lab _____

Peer _____

ACI _____

Epilepsy

Didactic _____

Lab _____

Peer _____

ACI _____

Syncope

Didactic _____

Lab _____

Peer _____

ACI _____

Reflex sympathetic dystrophy

Didactic _____

Lab _____

Peer _____

ACI _____

Meningitis

Didactic _____

Lab _____

Peer _____

ACI _____

Iron-deficiency anemia

Didactic _____

Lab _____

Peer _____

ACI _____

Sickle cell anemia

Didactic _____

Lab _____

Peer _____

ACI _____

Lyme disease

Didactic _____

Lab _____

Peer _____

ACI _____

COMMENTS

_____

_____

_____

_____

_____

_____

_____

Common Viral and Respiratory Tract Conditions and Disorders

Objective

Develop and demonstrate the skills necessary to evaluate, care for, and prevent common viral and respiratory tract conditions and disorders.

NATA Athletic Training Educational Competencies embedded in this module: AC-P4, MC-C2, MC-C3, MC-C7, MC-C8, MC-C9, MC-C16, MC-C19, MC-P4

Conditions and Disorders for This Module

- Common cold
- Influenza
- Laryngitis
- Pharyngitis
- Rhinitis
- Sinusitis
- Tetanus
- Tonsillitis
- Asthma
- Bronchitis
- Hyperventilation
- Hay fever
- Pneumonia
- Upper-respiratory infection

Competencies

1. Describe, with the use of pictures if necessary, the signs, symptoms, and predisposing conditions associated with the conditions and disorders listed in this module. Tell how each condition affects athletes' performances in American football, basketball, baseball and softball, track and field, and two other sports.

2. Explain, and demonstrate if possible, the appropriate management procedures for each condition. Explain the objectives and criteria for progressing for each step in the procedure.

3. Explain guidelines for participation (practice and games) for athletes with each condition.

4. Demonstrate or explain procedures for preventing each condition.

Proficiency Demonstration

1. Develop appropriate subject knowledge through coursework (C), verbal conversation (V), quizzes (Q), worksheets (W), or other approved activities (O).

2. Practice and reinforce the skills in clinical skills and laboratory courses.

3. Refine your skills by observing peer teachers and clinical instructors as they perform the skills (preferably on patients), discussing the competencies with peer teachers and clinical instructors, practicing alone and with others, and then demonstrating proficiency to a peer teacher.

4. Demonstrate your proficiency to an ACI.

APPROVED BY
(date and signature, and mode for didactic)

1-4. Complete competencies 1 through 4 for the following conditions and disorders.

Common cold
Didactic _____

Lab _____

Peer _____

ACI _____

Influenza
Didactic _____

Lab _____

Peer _____

ACI _____

Laryngitis
Didactic _____

Lab _____

Peer _____

ACI _____

Pharyngitis
Didactic _____

Lab _____

Peer _____

ACI _____

Rhinitis
Didactic _____

Lab _____

Peer _____

ACI _____

Sinusitis

Didactic _____

Lab _____

Peer _____

ACI _____

Tetanus

Didactic _____

Lab _____

Peer _____

ACI _____

Tonsillitis

Didactic _____

Lab _____

Peer _____

ACI _____

Asthma

Didactic _____

Lab _____

Peer _____

ACI _____

Bronchitis

Didactic _____

Lab _____

Peer _____

ACI _____

Hyperventilation

Didactic _____

Lab _____

Peer _____

ACI _____

Hay fever

Didactic _____

Lab _____

Peer _____

ACI _____

Pneumonia

Didactic _____

Lab _____

Peer _____

ACI _____

URI

Didactic _____

Lab _____

Peer _____

ACI _____

COMMENTS

_____

_____

_____

_____

_____

_____

_____

Common Cardiovascular and Gastrointestinal Tract Conditions and Disorders

Objective

Develop and demonstrate the skills necessary to evaluate, care for, and prevent common cardiovascular and gastrointestinal tract conditions and disorders.

NATA Athletic Training Educational Competencies embedded in this module: AC-P4. MC-C2, MC-C3, MC-C10, MC-C11, MC-C12, MC-C16, MC-C19, MC-P4

Conditions and Disorders for This Module

- Hypertension
- Hypotension
- Hypertrophic myocardiopathy
- Migraine headache
- Sudden death
- Appendicitis
- Colitis
- Constipation
- Diarrhea
- Esophageal reflux
- Gastritis
- Gastroenteritis
- Indigestion
- Ulcer
- Irritable bowel syndrome

Competencies

1. Describe, with the use of pictures if necessary, the signs, symptoms, and predisposing conditions associated with the conditions and disorders listed in this module. Tell how each condition affects athletes' performances in American football, basketball, baseball and softball, track and field, and two other sports.

2. Explain, and demonstrate if possible, the appropriate management procedures for each condition. Explain the objectives and criteria for progressing for each step in the procedure.

3. Explain guidelines for participation (practice and games) for athletes with each condition.

4. Demonstrate or explain procedures for preventing each condition.

Proficiency Demonstration

1. Develop appropriate subject knowledge through coursework (C), verbal conversation (V), quizzes (Q), worksheets (W), or other approved activities (O).

2. Practice and reinforce the skills in clinical skills and laboratory courses.

3. Refine your skills by observing peer teachers and clinical instructors as they perform the skills (preferably on patients), discussing the competencies with peer teachers and clinical instructors, practicing alone and with others, and then demonstrating proficiency to a peer teacher.

4. Demonstrate your proficiency to an ACI.

APPROVED BY
(date and signature, and mode for didactic)

1-4. Complete competencies 1 through 4 for the following conditions and disorders:

Hypertension

Didactic _____

Lab _____

Peer _____

ACI _____

Hypotension

Didactic _____

Lab _____

Peer _____

ACI _____

Hypertrophic myocardiopathy

Didactic _____

Lab _____

Peer _____

ACI _____

Migraine

Didactic _____

Lab _____

Peer _____

ACI _____

Sudden death

Didactic _____

Lab _____

Peer _____

ACI _____

Appendicitis

Didactic _____

Lab _____

Peer _____

ACI _____

Colitis

Didactic _____

Lab _____

Peer _____

ACI _____

Constipation

Didactic _____

Lab _____

Peer _____

ACI _____

Diarrhea

Didactic _____

Lab _____

Peer _____

ACI _____

Esophageal reflux

Didactic _____

Lab _____

Peer _____

ACI _____

Gastritis

Didactic _____

Lab _____

Peer _____

ACI _____

Gastroenteritis

Didactic _____

Lab _____

Peer _____

ACI _____

Indigestion

Didactic _____

Lab _____

Peer _____

ACI _____

Ulcer

Didactic _____

Lab _____

Peer _____

ACI _____

Irritable bowel syndrome

Didactic _____

Lab _____

Peer _____

ACI _____

COMMENTS

_____

_____

_____

_____

_____

_____

_____

Common Genitourinary, Gynecological, and Sexually Related Conditions, Disorders, and Diseases

Objective

Develop and demonstrate the skills necessary to evaluate, care for, and prevent common genitourinary, gynecological, and sexually related conditions, disorders, and diseases.

NATA Athletic Training Educational Competencies embedded in this module: MC-C2, MC-C3, MC-C14, MC-C16, MC-P4, AC-P4

Conditions and Disorders for This Module

- Kidney stones
- Spermatic cord torsion
- Candidiasis
- Urethritis
- Urinary tract infection
- Hydrocele
- Hemorrhoid
- Varicocele
- Amenorrhea
- Dysmenorrhea
- Oligomenorrhea
- Pelvic inflammatory disease
- Vaginitis
- HIV and acquired immunodeficiency syndrome (AIDS)
- Hepatitis
- Chlamydia
- Genital warts
- Gonorrhea
- Syphilis

Competencies

1. Describe, with the use of pictures if necessary, the signs, symptoms, and predisposing conditions associated with the conditions, diseases, and disorders listed in this module. Tell how each condition affects athletes' performances in American football, basketball, baseball and softball, track and field, and two other sports.

2. Explain, and demonstrate if possible, the appropriate management procedures for each condition listed. Explain the objectives and criteria for progressing for each step in the procedure.

3. Explain guidelines for participation (practice and games) for athletes with each condition.

4. Demonstrate or explain procedures for preventing each condition.

Proficiency Demonstration

1. Develop appropriate subject knowledge through coursework (C), verbal conversation (V), quizzes (Q), worksheets (W), or other approved activities (O).

2. Practice and reinforce the skills in clinical skills and laboratory courses.

3. Refine your skills by observing peer teachers and clinical instructors as they perform the skills (preferably on patients), discussing the competencies with peer teachers and clinical instructors, practicing alone and with others, and then demonstrating proficiency to a peer teacher.

4. Demonstrate your proficiency to an ACI.

APPROVED BY
(date and signature, and mode for didactic)

1-4. Complete competencies 1 through 4 for the following conditions, disorders, and diseases:

Kidney stones

Didactic _____

Lab _____

Peer _____

ACI _____

Spermatic cord torsion

Didactic _____

Lab _____

Peer _____

ACI _____

Candidiasis

Didactic _____

Lab _____

Peer _____

ACI _____

Urethritis

Didactic _____

Lab _____

Peer _____

ACI _____

Urinary tract infection

Didactic _____

Lab _____

Peer _____

ACI _____

Hydrocele

Didactic _____

Lab _____

Peer _____

ACI _____

Hemorrhoid

Didactic _____

Lab _____

Peer _____

ACI _____

Varicocele

Didactic _____

Lab _____

Peer _____

ACI _____

Amenorrhea

Didactic _____

Lab _____

Peer _____

ACI _____

Dysmenorrhea

Didactic _____

Lab _____

Peer _____

ACI _____

Oligomenorrhea

Didactic _____

Lab _____

Peer _____

ACI _____

Pelvic inflammatory disease

Didactic _____

Lab _____

Peer _____

ACI _____

Vaginitis

Didactic _____

Lab _____

Peer _____

ACI _____

HIV and AIDS

Didactic _____

Lab _____

Peer _____

ACI _____

Hepatitis

Didactic _____

Lab _____

Peer _____

ACI _____

Chlamydia

Didactic _____

Lab _____

Peer _____

ACI _____

Genital warts

Didactic _____

Lab _____

Peer _____

ACI _____

Gonorrhea

Didactic _____

Lab _____

Peer _____

ACI _____

Syphilis

Didactic _____

Lab _____

Peer _____

ACI _____

COMMENTS

_____

_____

_____

_____

Sudden Illnesses and Communicable Diseases

Objective

Develop and demonstrate the knowledge and skills to recognize and manage sudden illnesses and communicable diseases.

NATA Athletic Training Educational Competencies embedded in this module: AC-C27, AC-C28, AC-P2, AC-P3, AC-P4, MC-C1, MC-C2, MC-C3, MC-C18, PA-C1, PA-C5, PA-C6, RM-C2, RM-C6,

Sudden Illnesses and Communicable Diseases for This Module

- Shock
- Diabetic emergencies
- Seizures
- Fainting
- Closed head injuries
- Asthma
- Vocal cord dysfunction
- Allergic reactions and poisoning by the following:
  - Injection
  - Absorption
  - Inhalation
  - Ingestion
  - Substance use or misuse
- Infections
- Respiratory distress (adult, child, infant)
- Choking (adult, child, infant)
- Cardiac arrest and anomalies (adult, child, infant)
- Internal injuries
- Acute musculoskeletal injuries
- Spinal cord and peripheral nerve injuries
- Environmental illness and injuries (e.g., heat cramps, heat exhaustion, heat stroke, frostbite, hypothermia, drowning)

Competencies

1. Identify the signs, symptoms, and possible causes of the sudden illnesses and communicable diseases in the previous list.

2. Perform initial assessment procedures for the sudden illnesses and communicable diseases in the list.

3. Implement an emergency plan for the sudden illnesses and communicable diseases in the list.

4. Perform secondary assessment for the sudden illnesses and communicable diseases in the list.

5. Provide management procedures for the sudden illnesses and communicable diseases in the list.

Proficiency Demonstration

1. Develop appropriate subject knowledge through coursework (C), verbal conversation (V), quizzes (Q), worksheets (W), or other approved activities (O).

2. Practice and reinforce the skills in clinical skills and laboratory courses.

3. Refine your skills by observing peer teachers and clinical instructors as they perform the skills (preferably on patients), discussing the competencies with peer teachers and clinical instructors, practicing alone and with others, and then demonstrating proficiency to a peer teacher.

4. Demonstrate your proficiency to an ACI.

APPROVED BY
(date and signature, and mode for didactic)

1. Identifying signs, symptoms, and possible causes

Didactic _____

Lab _____

Peer _____

ACI _____

2. Performing initial assessment

Didactic _____

Lab _____

Peer _____

ACI _____

3. Emergency plan

Didactic _____

Lab _____

Peer _____

ACI _____

4. Secondary assessment

Didactic _____

Lab _____

Peer _____

ACI _____

5. Management procedures

Didactic _____

Lab _____

Peer _____

ACI _____

COMMENTS

_____

_____

_____

_____

_____

Therapeutic Modalities

Therapeutic modalities play an important role in the process of injury rehabilitation. Oftentimes, therapeutic modality use is referred to as *treatment* and can consist of thermal, electrical, magnetic, acoustic, and manual medicine applications. These treatments via therapeutic modalities are not to be viewed as standalone skills with specific start and end times; instead they should be considered as value-added components to the rehabilitation process.

Decisions regarding choice and timing of therapeutic modality treatment can increase or decrease healing time and affect the recovery of patients. Therapeutic modalities can facilitate and enhance therapeutic exercise activities and should be viewed as an important component of an AT's clinical skill set.

The following modules will provide opportunity to study, examine, review, and become clinically competent in the use of various therapeutic modality treatments and techniques. These modules will require an understanding of foundational principles and the physiological, pathological, and psychological processes of wound healing, tissue repair, and inflammation, as well as why these factors may or may not be helpful to the rehabilitation process. It will be necessary to actually perform the techniques or operate the equipment on patients prior to completion of the module.

Again, therapeutic modalities should not be used as isolated treatment; instead they should be viewed as integrated components of the rehabilitation process, which has the goal of returning function to a state of relative normalcy.

Therapeutic Modality Foundation

Objective

Develop an understanding of how the selection and application of therapeutic modalities during the treatment and rehabilitation phases of injury or illness affects the physiological, pathological, and psychological processes of inflammation, wound healing, and tissue repair.

NATA Athletic Training Educational Competencies embedded in this module: TM-C1, TM-C2, TM-C3, TM-C4, TM-C5 TM-C10, TM-C11

Competencies

1. Describe current pain control theories and how modality selection affects perception of pain.

2. Describe how various therapeutic modalities affect the following:
  a. Inflammatory process
  b. Wound healing or tissue repair
  c. Acute and chronic pain

3. Explain the following concepts as they apply to therapeutic modalities and identify the modalities that they concepts apply to:
  a. Electromagnetic spectra
  b. Acoustic spectra

4. Explain the basic concepts, principles, and terminology of electrical currents as they relate to therapeutic modalities and identify the modalities that they apply to.

5. Identify common pharmacological agents used with therapeutic modalities, and tell the specific modalities they are used with, their intended function, and their efficacy in meeting the intended function.

6. Discuss manufacturers', local, state, and federal operational standards for safe operation of therapeutic modalities.

7. Discuss manufacturers', local, state, and federal inspection and maintenance guidelines for therapeutic modalities.

Proficiency Demonstration

1. Develop appropriate subject knowledge through coursework (C), verbal conversation (V), quizzes (Q), worksheets (W), or other approved activities (O).

2. Practice and reinforce the skills in clinical skills and laboratory courses.

3. Refine your skills by observing peer teachers and clinical instructors as they perform the skills (preferably on patients), discussing the competencies with peer teachers and clinical instructors, practicing alone and with others, and then demonstrating proficiency to a peer teacher.

4. Demonstrate your proficiency to an ACI.

APPROVED BY
(date and signature, and mode for didactic)

1. Pain control

Didactic _____

Lab _____

Peer _____

ACI _____

2. Inflammation, wound healing, and acute or chronic pain

Didactic _____

Lab _____

Peer _____

ACI _____

3. Electromagnetic and acoustic spectra

Didactic _____

Lab _____

Peer _____

ACI _____

4. Electrical currents

Didactic _____

Lab _____

Peer _____

ACI _____

5. Pharmacological agents

Didactic _____

Lab _____

Peer _____

ACI _____

6. Operational standards

Didactic _____

Lab _____

Peer _____

ACI _____

7. Inspection and maintenance guidelines

Didactic _____

Lab _____

Peer _____

ACI _____

COMMENTS

_____

_____

_____

_____

_____

Whirlpool

Objective

Develop and demonstrate the skills necessary to use a whirlpool during sport injury rehabilitation.

NATA Athletic Training Educational Competencies embedded in this module: TM-C6, TM-C7, TM-C8, TM-C9, TM-P1, TM-P2, TM-P3, TM-P4, TM-P5, TM-P6, TM-CP1

Competencies

1. Define *whirlpool* and explain the following:
   a. Effects during and following application
   b. Advantages
   c. Disadvantages
   d. Indications
   e. Contraindications
   f. Precautions

2. Demonstrate and explain the following in relation to using a whirlpool to treat an upper-extremity injury, a lower-extremity injury, and general soreness:
   a. Preapplication procedures, including reevaluating the injury, evaluating the previous treatment, setting and evaluating goals, selecting the proper modality, and preparing the modality and patient
   b. Application procedures, including turn-on, adjustments, dosage, duration, and frequency of application
   c. Postapplication procedures, including patient and equipment cleanup, instructions to patient, and scheduling the next appointment

3. Demonstrate and explain maintenance and simple repair procedures for whirlpools.

4. Demonstrate recording of these treatments on athletic training clinic forms.

5. Properly treat a patient with a whirlpool following competencies 2 through 4.

Proficiency Demonstration

1. Develop appropriate subject knowledge through coursework (C), verbal conversation (V), quizzes (Q), worksheets (W), or other approved activities (O).

2. Practice and reinforce the skills in clinical skills and laboratory courses.

3. Refine your skills by observing peer teachers and clinical instructors as they perform the skills (preferably on patients), discussing the competencies with peer teachers and clinical instructors, practicing alone and with others, and then demonstrating proficiency to a peer teacher.

4. Demonstrate your proficiency to an ACI.

APPROVED BY
(date and signature, and mode for didactic)

1. Background
   Didactic _____
   Lab _____
   Peer _____
   ACI _____

2. Application
   Didactic _____
   Lab _____
   Peer _____
   ACI _____

3. Maintenance
   Didactic _____
   Lab _____
   Peer _____
   ACI _____

4. Recording
   Didactic _____
   Lab _____
   Peer _____
   ACI _____

5. Properly treating a patient
   Peer _____
   ACI _____

COMMENTS

_____

_____

_____

_____

Moist Hot Packs

Objective

Develop and demonstrate the skills necessary to use moist hot packs during sport injury rehabilitation.

NATA Athletic Training Educational Competencies embedded in this module: TM-C6, TM-C7, TM-C8, TM-C9, TM-P1, TM-P2, TM-P3, TM-P4, TM-P5, TM-P6, TM-CP1

Competencies

1. Define *hot pack* and explain the following:
   a. Effects during and following application
   b. Advantages
   c. Disadvantages
   d. Indications
   e. Contraindications
   f. Precautions

2. Demonstrate and explain the following in relation to using a moist hot pack for treating patellar tendinitis and neck soreness:
   a. Preapplication procedures, including reevaluating the injury, evaluating results of previous treatment, setting and evaluating goals, selecting proper modality, and preparing the modality and patient
   b. Application procedures, including turn-on, adjustments, dosage, duration, and frequency of application
   c. Postapplication procedures, including patient and equipment cleanup, instructions to the patient, and scheduling the next appointment

3. Demonstrate and explain maintenance and simple repair procedures for moist hot packs.

4. Demonstrate recording of these treatments on athletic training clinic forms.

5. Properly treat a patient with a moist heat pack following competencies 2 through 4.

Proficiency Demonstration

1. Develop appropriate subject knowledge through coursework (C), verbal conversation (V), quizzes (Q), worksheets (W), or other approved activities (O).

2. Practice and reinforce the skills in clinical skills and laboratory courses.

3. Refine your skills by observing peer teachers and clinical instructors as they perform the skills (preferably on patients), discussing the competencies with peer teachers and clinical instructors, practicing alone and with others, and then demonstrating proficiency to a peer teacher.

4. Demonstrate your proficiency to an ACI.

APPROVED BY
(date and signature, and mode for didactic)

1. Background
   Didactic _____
   Lab _____
   Peer _____
   ACI _____

2. Application
   Didactic _____
   Lab _____
   Peer _____
   ACI _____

3. Maintenance
   Didactic _____
   Lab _____
   Peer _____
   ACI _____

4. Recording
   Didactic _____
   Lab _____
   Peer _____
   ACI _____

5. Properly treating a patient
   Peer _____
   ACI _____

COMMENTS

_____

_____

_____

Paraffin Bath

Objective

Develop and demonstrate the skills necessary to use a paraffin bath during sport injury rehabilitation.

NATA Athletic Training Educational Competencies embedded in this module: TM-C6, TM-C7, TM-C8, TM-C9, TM-P1, TM-P2, TM-P3, TM-P4, TM-P5, TM-P6, TM-CP1

Competencies

1. Define *paraffin bath* and explain the following:
   a. Effects during and following application
   b. Advantages
   c. Disadvantages
   d. Indications
   e. Contraindications
   f. Precautions

2. Demonstrate and explain the following in relation to using a paraffin bath for treating a hand injury:
   a. Preapplication procedures, including reevaluating the injury, evaluating results of previous treatment, setting and evaluating goals, selecting proper modality, and preparing the modality and patient
   b. Application procedures, including turn-on, adjustments, dosage, duration, and frequency of application
   c. Postapplication procedures, including patient and equipment cleanup, instructions to patient, and scheduling the next appointment

3. Demonstrate and explain maintenance and simple repair procedures for paraffin baths.

4. Demonstrate recording of these treatments on athletic training clinic forms.

5. Properly treat a patient with a paraffin bath following competencies 2 through 4.

Proficiency Demonstration

1. Develop appropriate subject knowledge through coursework (C), verbal conversation (V), quizzes (Q), worksheets (W), or other approved activities (O).

2. Practice and reinforce the skills in clinical skills and laboratory courses.

3. Refine your skills by observing peer teachers and clinical instructors as they perform the skills (preferably on patients), discussing the competencies with peer teachers and clinical instructors, practicing alone and with others, and then demonstrating proficiency to a peer teacher.

4. Demonstrate your proficiency to an ACI.

APPROVED BY
(date and signature, and mode for didactic)

1. Background
   Didactic _____
   Lab _____
   Peer _____
   ACI _____

2. Application
   Didactic _____
   Lab _____
   Peer _____
   ACI _____

3. Maintenance
   Didactic _____
   Lab _____
   Peer _____
   ACI _____

4. Recording
   Didactic _____
   Lab _____
   Peer _____
   ACI _____

5. Properly treating a patient
   Peer _____
   ACI _____

COMMENTS

_____

_____

_____

_____

Cryotherapy

Objective

Develop and demonstrate the skills necessary to use cryotherapy during sport injury rehabilitation.

NATA Athletic Training Educational Competencies embedded in this module: TM-C6, TM-C7, TM-C8, TM-C9, TM-P1, TM-P2, TM-P3, TM-P4, TM-P5, TM-P6, TM-CP1

Competencies

1. Demonstrate and explain proper use of the following cryotherapy devices for treating an injury of your choice by performing the activities in the subsequent lettered list:

  Cold whirlpool treatment
  Controlled cold therapy unit
  Ice pack
  Vapocoolant spray
  Ice immersion
  Ice massage

  a. Define the modality and briefly explain its effects, advantages, disadvantages, indications, contraindications, and precautions.
  b. Demonstrate preapplication procedures, including reevaluating the injury, evaluating results of previous treatment, setting and evaluating goals, selecting proper modality, and preparing the modality and patient.
  c. Demonstrate and explain application procedures, including turn-on, adjustments, dosage, duration, and frequency of application.
  d. Demonstrate and explain postapplication procedures, including patient and equipment cleanup, instructions to the patient, and scheduling the next appointment.
  e. Demonstrate recording of these treatments on athletic training clinic forms.

2. Properly treat a patient with a cryotherapy device following the steps in competency 1.

Proficiency Demonstration

1. Develop appropriate subject knowledge through coursework (C), verbal conversation (V), quizzes (Q), worksheets (W), or other approved activities (O).

2. Practice and reinforce the skills in clinical skills and laboratory courses.

3. Refine your skills by observing peer teachers and clinical instructors as they perform the skills (preferably on patients), discussing the competencies with peer teachers and clinical instructors, practicing alone and with others, and then demonstrating proficiency to a peer teacher.

4. Demonstrate your proficiency to an ACI.

APPROVED BY
(date and signature, and mode for didactic)

Complete the activities in each competency for the following cryotherapy modalities.

1. Cold whirlpool
   Didactic _____
   Lab _____
   Peer _____
   ACI _____

2. Controlled cold therapy
   Didactic _____
   Lab _____
   Peer _____
   ACI _____

3. Ice packs
   Didactic _____
   Lab _____
   Peer _____
   ACI _____

4. Vapocoolant spray
   Didactic _____
   Lab _____
   Peer _____
   ACI _____

5. Ice immersion
   Didactic _____
   Lab _____
   Peer _____
   ACI _____

6. Ice massage

Didactic _____

Lab _____

Peer _____

ACI _____

7. Properly treating a patient

Peer _____

ACI _____

COMMENTS

_____

_____

_____

_____

_____

Cryokinetics

Objective

Develop and demonstrate the skills necessary to use cryokinetics during acute joint sprain rehabilitation.

NATA Athletic Training Educational Competencies embedded in this module: TM-C6, TM-C7, TM-C8, TM-C9, TM-P1, TM-P2, TM-P3, TM-P4, TM-P5, TM-P6, TM-CP1

Competencies

1. Define *cryokinetics* and explain the following:
   a. Effects
   b. Advantages
   c. Disadvantages
   d. Indications
   e. Contraindications
   f. Precautions

2. Demonstrate and explain cryokinetic treatments for an ankle sprain and for a finger sprain. Include the following for each treatment:
   a. Preapplication procedures, including reevaluating the injury, evaluating results of previous treatment, setting and evaluating goals, selecting proper modality and temperature, and preparing the modality and patient
   b. Application procedures, duration, and frequency of application
   c. Postapplication procedures, including patient and equipment cleanup, instructions to the patient, and scheduling the next appointment

3. Demonstrate recording of these treatments on athletic training clinic forms.

4. Properly treat a patient with cryokinetics following competencies 2 and 3.

Proficiency Demonstration

1. Develop appropriate subject knowledge through coursework (C), verbal conversation (V), quizzes (Q), worksheets (W), or other approved activities (O).

2. Practice and reinforce the skills in clinical skills and laboratory courses.

3. Refine your skills by observing peer teachers and clinical instructors as they perform the skills (preferably on patients), discussing the competencies with peer teachers and clinical instructors, practicing alone and with others, and then demonstrating proficiency to a peer teacher.

4. Demonstrate your proficiency to an ACI.

APPROVED BY
(date and signature, and mode for didactic)

1. Background
   Didactic _____
   Lab _____
   Peer _____
   ACI _____

2. Application
   Didactic _____
   Lab _____
   Peer _____
   ACI _____

3. Recording
   Didactic _____
   Lab _____
   Peer _____
   ACI _____

4. Properly treating a patient
   Peer _____
   ACI _____

COMMENTS

_____

_____

_____

_____

_____

_____

Cryostretch

Objective

Develop and demonstrate the skills necessary to use cryostretch during acute muscle strain rehabilitation.

NATA Athletic Training Educational Competencies embedded in this module: TM-C6, TM-C7, TM-C8, TM-C9, TM-P1, TM-P2, TM-P3, TM-P4, TM-P5, TM-P6, TM-CP1

Competencies

1. Define *cryostretch* and explain the following:
   a. Effects
   b. Advantages
   c. Disadvantages
   d. Indications
   e. Contraindications
   f. Precautions

2. Demonstrate and explain the following in relation to using cryostretch to treat a hamstring strain:
   a. Preapplication procedures, including reevaluating the injury, evaluating results of previous treatment, setting and evaluating goals, selecting proper modality, and preparing the modality and patient
   b. Application procedures, duration, and frequency of application
   c. Postapplication procedures, including patient and equipment cleanup, instructions to the patient, and scheduling the next appointment

3. Demonstrate recording of these treatments on athletic training clinic forms.

4. Properly treat a patient with a cryostretch following competencies 2 and 3.

Proficiency Demonstration

1. Develop appropriate subject knowledge through coursework (C), verbal conversation (V), quizzes (Q), worksheets (W), or other approved activities (O).

2. Practice and reinforce the skills in clinical skills and laboratory courses.

3. Refine your skills by observing peer teachers and clinical instructors as they perform the skills (preferably on patients), discussing the competencies with peer teachers and clinical instructors, practicing alone and with others, and then demonstrating proficiency to a peer teacher.

4. Demonstrate your proficiency to an ACI.

APPROVED BY
(date and signature, and mode for didactic)

1. Background
   Didactic _____
   Lab _____
   Peer _____
   ACI _____

2. Application
   Didactic _____
   Lab _____
   Peer _____
   ACI _____

3. Recording
   Didactic _____
   Lab _____
   Peer _____
   ACI _____

4. Properly treating a patient
   Peer _____
   ACI _____

COMMENTS

_____

_____

_____

_____

_____

_____

Lymphedema Devices

Objective

Develop and demonstrate the skills necessary to use a lymphedema device during sport injury rehabilitation.

NATA Athletic Training Educational Competencies embedded in this module: TM-C6, TM-C7, TM-C8, TM-C9, TM-P1, TM-P2, TM-P3, TM-P4, TM-P5, TM-P6, TM-CP1

Competencies

1. Define *lymphedema device* and explain the following:
   a. Therapeutic effects
   b. Advantages
   c. Disadvantages
   d. Indications
   e. Contraindications
   f. Precautions

2. Demonstrate and explain the following in relation to treating a hand contusion with a lymphedema device:
   a. Preapplication procedures, including reevaluating the injury, evaluating results of previous treatment, setting and evaluating goals, selecting proper modality, and preparing the modality and patient
   b. Application procedures, including turn-on, adjustments, dosage, duration, and frequency of application
   c. Postapplication procedures, including patient and equipment cleanup, instructions to the patient, and scheduling the next appointment

3. Demonstrate and explain maintenance and simple repair procedures for lymphedema devices.

4. Demonstrate recording of lymphedema device treatments on athletic training clinic forms.

5. Properly treat a patient with a lymphedema device following competencies 2 through 4.

Proficiency Demonstration

1. Develop appropriate subject knowledge through coursework (C), verbal conversation (V), quizzes (Q), worksheets (W), or other approved activities (O).

2. Practice and reinforce the skills in clinical skills and laboratory courses.

3. Refine your skills by observing peer teachers and clinical instructors as they perform the skills (preferably on patients), discussing the competencies with peer teachers and clinical instructors, practicing alone and with others, and then demonstrating proficiency to a peer teacher.

4. Demonstrate your proficiency to an ACI.

APPROVED BY
(date and signature, and mode for didactic)

1. Background
   Didactic _____
   Lab _____
   Peer _____
   ACI _____

2. Application
   Didactic _____
   Lab _____
   Peer _____
   ACI _____

3. Maintenance
   Didactic _____
   Lab _____
   Peer _____
   ACI _____

4. Recording
   Didactic _____
   Lab _____
   Peer _____
   ACI _____

5. Properly treating a patient
   Peer _____
   ACI _____

COMMENTS

_____

_____

_____

_____

Ultrasound

Objective

Develop and demonstrate the skills necessary to use ultrasound during sport injury rehabilitation.

NATA Athletic Training Educational Competencies embedded in this module: TM-C2, TM-C3, TM-C5, TM-C6, TM-C7, TM-C8, TM-C9, TM-P1, TM-P1, TM-P2, TM-P3, TM-P4, TM-P5, TM-P6, TM-CP1

Competencies

1. Define and briefly explain the following:
   a. Thermal ultrasound treatment
   b. Nonthermal ultrasound treatment
   c. Combination electrical stimulation and ultrasound treatment
   d. Phonophoresis treatment
   e. Indirect application of ultrasound treatment (underwater, bladder)

2. For each of the ultrasound types in competency 1, explain the following:
   a. Therapeutic effects
   b. Advantages
   c. Disadvantages
   d. Indications
   e. Contraindications
   f. Precautions

3. For each of the ultrasound types in competency 1, demonstrate and explain the following for treating an injury of your choice:
   a. Preapplication procedures, including reevaluating the injury, evaluating results of previous treatment, setting and evaluating goals, selecting proper modality, and preparing the modality and patient
   b. Application procedures, including turn-on, adjustments, dosage, duration, and frequency of application
   c. Postapplication procedures, including patient and equipment cleanup, instructions to the patient, and scheduling the next appointment

4. Demonstrate and explain maintenance and simple repair procedures for ultrasound machines.

5. Demonstrate recording of ultrasound treatments on athletic training clinic forms.

6. Properly treat a patient with ultrasound following competencies 2 through 5.

Proficiency Demonstration

1. Develop appropriate subject knowledge through coursework (C), verbal conversation (V), quizzes (Q), worksheets (W), or other approved activities (O).

2. Practice and reinforce the skills in clinical skills and laboratory courses.

3. Refine your skills by observing peer teachers and clinical instructors as they perform the skills (preferably on patients), discussing the competencies with peer teachers and clinical instructors, practicing alone and with others, and then demonstrating proficiency to a peer teacher.

4. Demonstrate your proficiency to an ACI.

APPROVED BY
(date and signature, and mode for didactic)

1-3. Complete competencies 1-3 for the following:

Thermal ultrasound

Didactic _____

Lab _____

Peer _____

ACI _____

Nonthermal ultrasound

Didactic _____

Lab _____

Peer _____

ACI _____

Combination electrical stimulation and ultrasound

Didactic _____

Lab _____

Peer _____

ACI _____

Phonophoresis

Didactic _____

Lab _____

Peer _____

ACI _____

Indirect application

Didactic _____

Lab _____

Peer _____

ACI _____

4. Maintenance

Didactic _____

Lab _____

Peer _____

ACI _____

5. Recording

Didactic _____

Lab _____

Peer _____

ACI _____

6. Properly treating a patient

Peer _____

ACI _____

COMMENTS

_____

_____

_____

_____

_____

_____

_____

_____

_____

Pulsed Shortwave Diathermy

Objective

Develop and demonstrate the skills necessary to use diathermy during sport injury rehabilitation.

NATA Athletic Training Educational Competencies embedded in this module: TM-C2, TM-C3, TM-C5, TM-C6, TM-C7, TM-C8, TM-C9, TM-P1, TM-P1, TM-P2, TM-P3, TM-P4, TM-P5, TM-P6, TM-CP1

Competencies

1. Define *pulsed shortwave diathermy* and explain the following:
   a. Therapeutic effects during and following application
   b. Advantages
   c. Disadvantages
   d. Indications
   e. Contraindications
   f. Precautions

2. Demonstrate and explain the following for treating an injury of your choice with pulsed shortwave diathermy:
   a. Preapplication procedures, including reevaluating the injury, evaluating results of previous treatment, setting and evaluating goals, selecting proper modality, and preparing the modality and patient
   b. Application procedures, including turn-on, adjustments, dosage, duration, and frequency of application
   c. Postapplication procedures, including patient and equipment cleanup, instructions to the patient, and scheduling the next appointment

3. Demonstrate and explain maintenance and simple repair procedures for pulsed shortwave diathermy machines.

4. Demonstrate recording of pulsed shortwave diathermy treatments on athletic training clinic forms.

5. Properly treat a patient with pulsed shortwave diathermy following competencies 2 through 4.

Proficiency Demonstration

1. Develop appropriate subject knowledge through coursework (C), verbal conversation (V), quizzes (Q), worksheets (W), or other approved activities (O).

2. Practice and reinforce the skills in clinical skills and laboratory courses.

3. Refine your skills by observing peer teachers and clinical instructors as they perform the skills (pref-erably on patients), discussing the competencies with peer teachers and clinical instructors, practicing alone and with others, and then demonstrating proficiency to a peer teacher.

4. Demonstrate your proficiency to an ACI.

APPROVED BY
(date and signature, and mode for didactic)

1. Background
   Didactic _____
   Lab _____
   Peer _____
   ACI _____

2. Application
   Didactic _____
   Lab _____
   Peer _____
   ACI _____

3. Maintenance
   Didactic _____
   Lab _____
   Peer _____
   ACI _____

4. Recording
   Didactic _____
   Lab _____
   Peer _____
   ACI _____

5. Properly treating a patient
   Peer _____
   ACI _____

COMMENTS

_____

_____

_____

Electrical Stimulation

Objective

Develop and demonstrate the skills necessary to use electrical stimulation during sport injury rehabilitation.

NATA Athletic Training Educational Competencies embedded in this module: TM-C2, TM-C3, TM-C5, TM-C6, TM-C7, TM-C8, TM-C9, TM-P1, TM-P1, TM-P2, TM-P3, TM-P4, TM-P5, TM-P6, TM-CP1

Competencies

1. Briefly explain electrical stimulation and its use, including the type of electrical stimulator and the specific settings you would use to achieve the following:
   a. Sensory-level pain control
   b. Noxious-level pain control
   c. Motor-level pain control
   d. Muscle reeducation
   e. Muscle pumping
   f. Muscle atrophy retardation
   g. Acute edema reduction
   h. Muscle splinting and spasm reduction
   i. Iontophoresis

2. For each of the goals of electrical stimulation in competency 1, demonstrate and explain the following, using the proper electrical simulator to treat an injury of your choice:
   a. Preapplication procedures, including reevaluating the injury, evaluating results of previous treatment, setting and evaluating goals, selecting proper modality, and preparing the modality and patient
   b. Application procedures, including turn-on, adjustments, dosage, duration, and frequency of application
   c. Postapplication procedures, including patient and equipment cleanup, instructions to the patient, and scheduling the next appointment
   d. Maintenance and simple repair procedures for electrical muscle stimulation machines
   e. Proper recording of electrical stimulation treatments on athletic training clinic forms

3. For each of the following electrical stimulation units not used in competency 2, demonstrate and explain its use to achieve one of the goals in competency 1.
   a. Monophasic stimulator (e.g., high-volt stimulation)

   b. Biphasic stimulator (e.g., transcutaneous electrical nerve stimulation [TENS] and neuromuscular electrical stimulation [NMES])
   c. Direct current (e.g., iontophoresis)
   d. Alternating current (e.g., interferential, NMES)
   e. Multifunction electrical stimulation devices

4. Properly treat a patient with electrical stimulation following competencies 2 and 3.

Proficiency Demonstration

1. Develop appropriate subject knowledge through coursework (C), verbal conversation (V), quizzes (Q), worksheets (W), or other approved activities (O).

2. Practice and reinforce the skills in clinical skills and laboratory courses.

3. Refine your skills by observing peer teachers and clinical instructors as they perform the skills (preferably on patients), discussing the competencies with peer teachers and clinical instructors, practicing alone and with others, and then demonstrating proficiency to a peer teacher.

4. Demonstrate your proficiency to an ACI.

APPROVED BY
(date and signature, and mode for didactic)

1-3. Complete competencies 1 through 3 for the following:

Sensory-level pain control

Didactic _____

Lab _____

Peer _____

ACI _____

Noxious-level pain control

Didactic _____

Lab _____

Peer _____

ACI _____

Motor-level pain control

Didactic _____

Lab _____

Peer _____

ACI _____

Muscle reeducation

Didactic _____

Lab _____

Peer _____

ACI _____

Muscle pumping

Didactic _____

Lab _____

Peer _____

ACI _____

Muscle atrophy retardation

Didactic _____

Lab _____

Peer _____

ACI _____

Acute edema reduction

Didactic _____

Lab _____

Peer _____

ACI _____

Muscle splinting and spasm reduction

Didactic _____

Lab _____

Peer _____

ACI _____

Iontophoresis

Didactic _____

Lab _____

Peer _____

ACI _____

Monophasic stimulator

Didactic _____

Lab _____

Peer _____

ACI _____

Biphasic stimulator

Didactic _____

Lab _____

Peer _____

ACI _____

Direct current

Didactic _____

Lab _____

Peer _____

ACI _____

Alternating current

Didactic _____

Lab _____

Peer _____

ACI _____

Multifunction electrical stimulation devices

Didactic _____

Lab _____

Peer _____

ACI _____

4. Properly treating a patient

Sensory-level pain control

Peer _____

ACI _____

COMMENTS

_____

_____

_____

_____

_____

Therapeutic Massage

Objective

Develop and demonstrate the skills necessary to use massage during sport injury rehabilitation.

NATA Athletic Training Educational Competencies embedded in this module: EX-C5, TM-C6, TM-C7, TM-C8, TM-C9, TM-P1, TM-P2, TM-P3, TM-P4, TM-P5, TM-P6

Competencies

1. Briefly explain and differentiate among the following massage strokes:
- a. Effleurage
- b. Petrissage
- c. Friction (circular, transverse)
- d. Tapotement
- e. Vibration
- f. Myofascial release techniques

2. For each of the massage strokes in competency 1, explain the following:
- – Therapeutic effects both during and after massage
- – Advantages
- – Disadvantages
- – Indications
- – Contraindications
- – Precautions

3. Demonstrate each of the massage strokes in competency 1.

4. Demonstrate and explain an overall or integrated therapeutic massage treatment, including the following:
- a. Preapplication procedures, including reevaluating the injury, evaluating results of previous treatment, setting and evaluating goals, selecting proper modality, and preparing the patient
- b. Application procedures, including types and sequence of strokes, adjustments, duration, and frequency of application
- c. Postapplication procedures, including patient and equipment cleanup, instructions to the patient, and scheduling the next appointment
- d. Recording of massage treatments on athletic training clinic forms

5. Properly treat a patient with massage following competencies 2 through 4.

Proficiency Demonstration

1. Develop appropriate subject knowledge through coursework (C), verbal conversation (V), quizzes (Q), worksheets (W), or other approved activities (O).

2. Practice and reinforce the skills in clinical skills and laboratory courses.

3. Refine your skills by observing peer teachers and clinical instructors as they perform the skills (preferably on patients), discussing the competencies with peer teachers and clinical instructors, practicing alone and with others, and then demonstrating proficiency to a peer teacher.

4. Demonstrate your proficiency to an ACI.

APPROVED BY
(date and signature, and mode for didactic)

1-3. Complete competencies 1 through 3 for the following massage strokes:

Effleurage

Didactic _____

Lab _____

Peer _____

ACI _____

Petrissage

Didactic _____

Lab _____

Peer _____

ACI _____

Friction (circular, transverse)

Didactic _____

Lab _____

Peer _____

ACI _____

Tapotement

Didactic _____

Lab _____

Peer _____

ACI _____

Vibration

Didactic _____

Lab _____

Peer _____

ACI _____

Myofascial release techniques

Didactic _____

Lab _____

Peer _____

ACI _____

4. Overall massage

Didactic _____

Lab _____

Peer _____

ACI _____

5. Properly treating a patient

Peer _____

ACI _____

COMMENTS

_____

_____

_____

_____

_____

_____

Traction

Objective

Develop and demonstrate the skills necessary to use traction during sport injury rehabilitation.

NATA Athletic Training Educational Competencies embedded in this module: EX-C5, TM-C6, TM-C7, TM-C8, TM-C9, TM-P1, TM-P2, TM-P3, TM-P4, TM-P5, TM-P6

Competencies

1. Briefly explain and differentiate among the following:
   a. Mechanical traction
   b. Manual traction
   c. Positional traction

2. For each type of traction in competency 1, explain the following:
   – Therapeutic effects
   – Advantages
   – Disadvantages
   – Indications
   – Contraindications
   – Precautions

3. For each type of traction in competency 1, demonstrate and explain the following:
   – Preapplication procedures, including reevaluating the injury, evaluating results of previous treatment, setting and evaluating goals, selecting proper modality, and preparing the modality and patient
   – Application procedures, including turn-on, adjustments, dosage, duration, and frequency of application
   – Postapplication procedures, including patient and equipment cleanup, instructions to the patient, and scheduling the next appointment

4. Demonstrate and explain maintenance and simple repair procedures for traction devices.

5. Demonstrate recording of traction treatments on athletic training clinic forms.

6. Properly apply traction to a patient following competencies 3 through 5.

Proficiency Demonstration

1. Develop appropriate subject knowledge through coursework (C), verbal conversation (V), quizzes (Q), worksheets (W), or other approved activities (O).

2. Practice and reinforce the skills in clinical skills and laboratory courses.

3. Refine your skills by observing peer teachers and clinical instructors as they perform the skills (preferably on patients), discussing the competencies with peer teachers and clinical instructors, practicing alone and with others, and then demonstrating proficiency to a peer teacher.

4. Demonstrate your proficiency to an ACI.

APPROVED BY
(date and signature, and mode for didactic)

1-3. Complete competencies 1 through 3 for the following types of traction:

Mechanical traction

Didactic _____

Lab _____

Peer _____

ACI _____

Manual traction

Didactic _____

Lab _____

Peer _____

ACI _____

Positional traction

Didactic _____

Lab _____

Peer _____

ACI _____

4. Maintenance

Didactic _____

Lab _____

Peer _____

ACI _____

5. Recording

Didactic _____

Lab _____

Peer _____

ACI _____

6. Properly treating a patient

Peer _____

ACI _____

COMMENTS

_____

_____

_____

_____

_____

Therapeutic Exercise

The most visible component of the rehabilitation process is often therapeutic exercise. It is the component that many people equate with the rehabilitation process, and it is known for being physically difficult, challenging, and time consuming. Though it is true that the techniques and strategies for stretching, lifting, exercising, conditioning, training, and so on are both demanding and important, the overall rehabilitation outcome might be unfavorable if the foundation for this process is not initiated with appropriate acute care, assessment, and modality treatment. Improper acute care and treatment can slow down or even prevent a return to former capabilities regardless of therapeutic exercises.

ATs must develop the knowledge and clinical skills to apply therapeutic exercise. Because physical activity requires multiple musculoskeletal attributes and systemic functions, various therapeutic exercises have been developed to address each of these areas. Use of therapeutic exercise is important for restoring and developing ROM, strength, balance, agility, cardiorespiratory fitness, muscular endurance, and activity-specific skills.

Each type of therapeutic exercise may include multiple activities due to the complex nature of physical movement. Performance of multiple activities from several categories of therapeutic exercise may have to be combined during an exercise session to address the total needs of the patient.

The list of activities that address the goal of each therapeutic exercise category is large and ever expanding based on the creativity and ingenuity of the AT. Students must first understand the purpose and goals for each therapeutic exercise category and then examine which individual training exercises and activities meet those objectives.

In the following modules, the student is expected to review and develop clinical competence in performing the exercise prescription skills needed for effective rehabilitation of injuries and illnesses affecting the musculoskeletal, cardiovascular, and neurological systems of an active population.

Range-of-Motion and Flexibility Exercises

Objective

Develop and demonstrate the skills necessary to use therapeutic exercise to improve ROM and flexibility during sport injury rehabilitation.

NATA Athletic Training Educational Competencies embedded in this module: EX-C1, EX-C2, EX-C3, EX-C4, EX-C5, EX-C6, EX-C7, EX-P1, EX-P2, EX-P4, EX-P5, EX-P6, EX-P7, EX-CP1, RM-P1, RM-P2, RM-CP1

Competencies

1. Discuss the role of improving ROM and flexibility during sport injury rehabilitation, including when it should be performed during the rehabilitation process.

2. Discuss the difference between anatomic and functional ROM and give examples of each.

3. Discuss the role of joint mobilization in increasing ROM and flexibility.

4. Demonstrate use of a goniometer to measure ROM at three joints.

5. Demonstrate use of the following types of therapeutic exercise for improving upper-extremity ROM and flexibility:
   a. Passive ROM
   b. Active ROM
   c. Active-assisted ROM, by performing the elements of therapeutic exercise in this list:
      – Position the patient.
      – Stabilize the patient during repetitions.
      – Demonstrate and instruct proper execution of repetitions (form, timing, control).
      – Explain how and when to adjust the exercise.
      – Demonstrate ways an athlete can cheat while performing the exercise.
      – Outline safety factors for the athlete and yourself.
      – Demonstrate how to record the results of the therapeutic exercise session.

6. Demonstrate use of the following types of therapeutic exercise for improving lower-extremity ROM and flexibility by performing the elements of therapeutic exercise in the list in competency 5:
   a. Passive ROM
   b. Active ROM
   c. Active-assisted ROM

7. Demonstrate use of the following types of therapeutic exercise for improving trunk extremity ROM and flexibility by performing the elements of therapeutic exercise in the list in competency 5:
   a. Passive ROM
   b. Active ROM
   c. Active-assisted ROM

8. Demonstrate use of the following types of therapeutic exercise for improving cervical spine ROM and flexibility by performing the elements of therapeutic exercise in the list in competency 5:
   a. Passive ROM
   b. Active ROM
   c. Active-assisted ROM

Proficiency Demonstration

1. Develop appropriate subject knowledge through coursework (C), verbal conversation (V), quizzes (Q), worksheets (W), or other approved activities (O).

2. Practice and reinforce the skills in clinical skills and laboratory courses.

3. Refine your skills by observing peer teachers and clinical instructors as they perform the skills (preferably on patients), discussing the competencies with peer teachers and clinical instructors, practicing alone and with others, and then demonstrating proficiency to a peer teacher.

4. Demonstrate your proficiency to an ACI.

APPROVED BY
(date and signature, and mode for didactic)

1. Background
   Didactic _____
   Lab _____
   Peer _____
   ACI _____

2. Anatomic versus functional ROM
   Didactic _____
   Lab _____
   Peer _____
   ACI _____

3. Role of joint mobilization
   Didactic _____
   Lab _____
   Peer _____
   ACI _____

4. Goniometer

Didactic _____

Lab _____

Peer _____

ACI _____

5a. Upper extremity—passive ROM

Didactic _____

Lab _____

Peer _____

ACI _____

5b. Upper extremity—active ROM

Didactic _____

Lab _____

Peer _____

ACI _____

5c. Upper extremity—active-assisted ROM

Didactic _____

Lab _____

Peer _____

ACI _____

6a. Lower extremity—passive ROM

Didactic _____

Lab _____

Peer _____

ACI _____

6b. Lower extremity—active ROM

Didactic _____

Lab _____

Peer _____

ACI _____

6c. Lower extremity—active-assisted ROM

Didactic _____

Lab _____

Peer _____

ACI _____

7a. Trunk—passive ROM

Didactic _____

Lab _____

Peer _____

ACI _____

7b. Trunk—active ROM

Didactic _____

Lab _____

Peer _____

ACI _____

7c. Trunk—active-assisted ROM

Didactic _____

Lab _____

Peer _____

ACI _____

8a. Cervical spine—passive ROM

Didactic _____

Lab _____

Peer _____

ACI _____

8b. Cervical spine—active ROM

Didactic _____

Lab _____

Peer _____

ACI _____

8c. Cervical spine—active-assisted ROM

Didactic _____

Lab _____

Peer _____

ACI _____

COMMENTS

_____

_____

_____

Joint Mobilization

Objective

Develop and demonstrate the skills necessary to use mobilization during sport injury rehabilitation.

NATA Athletic Training Educational Competencies embedded in this module: DI-C5, EX-C1, EX-C2, EX-C3, EX-C4, EX-C5, EX-C6, EX-C7, EX-P1, EX-P2, EX-P4, EX-P5, EX-P6, EX-P7, EX-CP1, RM-P1, RM-P2, RM-CP1

Competencies

1. Define and briefly explain mobilization, including the following:
  a. Therapeutic effects
  b. Advantages
  c. Disadvantages
  d. Indications
  e. Contraindications
  f. Precautions

2. Define and demonstrate the following:
  a. Loose- and close-packed positions
  b. Joint play
  c. Roll, glide, spin
  d. Concave and convex rules
  e. Long-axis distraction
  f. Glides (e.g., anterior–posterior, superior–inferior)

3. Define and demonstrate grades I through IV of mobilization as defined by Maitland by doing the following:
  – Preapplication procedures, including reevaluating the injury, evaluating results of previous treatment, setting and evaluating goals, selecting proper modality, and preparing the patient
  – Application procedures, hand placement, force, repetitions, adjustments, duration, and frequency of application
  – Postapplication procedures, including patient cleanup, instructions to the patient, and scheduling the next appointment
  – Proper recording of joint mobilization treatments on athletic training clinic forms

4. Define and demonstrate self-mobilization for a body part of your choice.

Proficiency Demonstration

1. Develop appropriate subject knowledge through coursework (C), verbal conversation (V), quizzes (Q), worksheets (W), or other approved activities (O).

2. Practice and reinforce the skills in clinical skills and laboratory courses.

3. Refine your skills by observing peer teachers and clinical instructors as they perform the skills (preferably on patients), discussing the competencies with peer teachers and clinical instructors, practicing alone and with others, and then demonstrating proficiency to a peer teacher.

4. Demonstrate your proficiency to an ACI.

APPROVED BY
(date and signature, and mode for didactic)

1. Background
Didactic _____
Lab _____
Peer _____
ACI _____

2a. Loose- and close-packed positions
Didactic _____
Lab _____
Peer _____
ACI _____

2b. Joint play
Didactic _____
Lab _____
Peer _____
ACI _____

2c. Roll, glide, spin
Didactic _____
Lab _____
Peer _____
ACI _____

2d. Concave and convex rules
Didactic _____
Lab _____
Peer _____
ACI _____

2e. Long-axis distraction

Didactic _____

Lab _____

Peer _____

ACI _____

2f. Glides (anterior–posterior, superior–inferior)

Didactic _____

Lab _____

Peer _____

ACI _____

3. Maitland mobilization grades—I through IV

Didactic _____

Lab _____

Peer _____

ACI _____

4. Self-mobilization

Didactic _____

Lab _____

Peer _____

ACI _____

COMMENTS

_____

_____

_____

_____

_____

_____

_____

Isometric Resistance Exercises

Objective

Develop and demonstrate the skills necessary to use isometric resistance exercises during sport injury rehabilitation.

NATA Athletic Training Educational Competencies embedded in this module: EX-C1, EX-C2, EX-C3, EX-C4, EX-C5, EX-C6, EX-C7, EX-P1, EX-P2, EX-P4, EX-P5, EX-P6, EX-P7, EX-CP1, RM-P1, RM-P2, RM-CP1

Competencies

1. Discuss isometric resistance, how it is developed, the equipment needed, and its similarities to and differences from isotonic and isokinetic resistance.

2. Demonstrate use of isometrics for strengthening the following:
   a. Lower extremity
   b. Upper extremity
   c. Cervical spine
   d. Trunk and torso, by performing the elements of therapeutic exercise in this list:
   – Set up the equipment.
   – Position the patient.
   – Stabilize the patient during repetitions.
   – Demonstrate and instruct proper execution of repetitions (form, timing, control).
   – Explain how and when to adjust the equipment.
   – Demonstrate ways an athlete can cheat on the equipment.
   – Outline safety factors for the athlete and yourself.
   – Demonstrate how to record the results of the therapeutic exercise session.
   – Demonstrate and explain maintenance and simple repair procedures for the equipment.

Proficiency Demonstration

1. Develop appropriate subject knowledge through coursework (C), verbal conversation (V), quizzes (Q), worksheets (W), or other approved activities (O).

2. Practice and reinforce the skills in clinical skills and laboratory courses.

3. Refine your skills by observing peer teachers and clinical instructors as they perform the skills (preferably on patients), discussing the competencies with peer teachers and clinical instructors, practicing alone and with others, and then demonstrating proficiency to a peer teacher.

4. Demonstrate your proficiency to an ACI.

APPROVED BY
(date and signature, and mode for didactic)

1. Background
   Didactic _____
   Lab _____
   Peer _____
   ACI _____

2a. Lower extremity
   Didactic _____
   Lab _____
   Peer _____
   ACI _____

2b. Upper extremity
   Didactic _____
   Lab _____
   Peer _____
   ACI _____

2c. Cervical spine
   Didactic _____
   Lab _____
   Peer _____
   ACI _____

2d. Trunk and torso
   Didactic _____
   Lab _____
   Peer _____
   ACI _____

COMMENTS

_____

_____

_____

_____

Isotonic Strength Training Devices

Objective

Develop and demonstrate the skills necessary to use isotonic devices to develop strength during sport injury rehabilitation.

NATA Athletic Training Educational Competencies embedded in this module: EX-C1, EX-C2, EX-C3, EX-C4, EX-C5, EX-C6, EX-C7, EX-P1, EX-P2, EX-P3, EX-P4, EX-P5, EX-P6, EX-P7, EX-CP1, RM-P1, RM-P2, RM-CP1

Competencies

1. Discuss isotonic resistance, how it is developed, the equipment needed, and its similarities to and differences from isometric and isokinetic resistance.

2. Demonstrate use of isotonic weight training equipment for strengthening the following:
   a. Knee and thigh (using a knee flexion and extension machine)
   b. Overall legs (leg press or squat)
   c. Shoulder (abduction and internal and external rotation)
   d. Trunk and torso
   e. Cervical spine, by performing the elements of therapeutic exercise in this list:
      – Set up the equipment.
      – Position the patient.
      – Stabilize the patient during repetitions.
      – Demonstrate proper execution of repetitions (form, timing, control).
      – Explain how and when to adjust the equipment.
      – Demonstrate ways an athlete can cheat on the equipment.
      – Outline safety factors for the athlete and yourself.
      – Demonstrate how to record results.
      – Demonstrate and explain maintenance and simple repair procedures.

Proficiency Demonstration

1. Develop appropriate subject knowledge through coursework (C), verbal conversation (V), quizzes (Q), worksheets (W), or other approved activities (O).

2. Practice and reinforce the skills in clinical skills and laboratory courses.

3. Refine your skills by observing peer teachers and clinical instructors as they perform the skills (preferably on patients), discussing the competencies with peer teachers and clinical instructors, practicing alone and with others, and then demonstrating proficiency to a peer teacher.

4. Demonstrate your proficiency to an ACI.

APPROVED BY
(date and signature, and mode for didactic)

1. Background
   Didactic _____
   Lab _____
   Peer _____
   ACI _____

2a. Knee and thigh (using a knee flexion and extension machine)
   Didactic _____
   Lab _____
   Peer _____
   ACI _____

2b. Overall legs (leg press or squat)
   Didactic _____
   Lab _____
   Peer _____
   ACI _____

2c. Shoulder (abduction and internal and external rotation)
   Didactic _____
   Lab _____
   Peer _____
   ACI _____

2d. Trunk and torso
   Didactic _____
   Lab _____
   Peer _____
   ACI _____

2e. Cervical spine

Didactic _____

Lab

Peer_____

ACI _____

COMMENTS

_____

_____

_____

Daily Adjustable Progressive Resistive Exercise

Objective

Develop and demonstrate the skills necessary to use the daily adjustable progressive exercise (DAPRE) technique for evaluating and redeveloping strength during sport injury rehabilitation.

NATA Athletic Training Educational Competencies embedded in this module: EX-C1, EX-C2, EX-C3, EX-C4, EX-C5, EX-C6, EX-C7, EX-P1, EX-P2, EX-P3, EX-P4, EX-P5, EX-P6, EX-P7, EX-CP1, RM-P1, RM-P2, RM-CP1

Competencies

1. Define *DAPRE* and explain the following:
   a. Effects
   b. Advantages
   c. Disadvantages
   d. Indications
   e. Contraindications
   f. Precautions

2. Explain why the DAPRE technique can only be used with isotonic and isometric equipment.

3. Explain the role of verbal encouragement during DAPRE and demonstrate how to verbally encourage athletes to perform to their fullest.

4. Demonstrate and explain use of the DAPRE technique for the following:
   a. Knee strength development
   b. Ankle strength development
   c. Shoulder strength development

5. Demonstrate and explain how to use the DAPRE technique for strength maintenance.

6. Demonstrate and explain how to use the DAPRE technique to evaluate strength maintenance.

7. Demonstrate proper recording of these treatments on athletic training clinic forms.

Proficiency Demonstration

1. Develop appropriate subject knowledge through coursework (C), verbal conversation (V), quizzes (Q), worksheets (W), or other approved activities (O).

2. Practice and reinforce the skills in clinical skills and laboratory courses.

3. Refine your skills by observing peer teachers and clinical instructors as they perform the skills (preferably on patients), discussing the competencies with peer teachers and clinical instructors, practicing alone and with others, and then demonstrating proficiency to a peer teacher.

4. Demonstrate your proficiency to an ACI.

APPROVED BY
(date and signature, and mode for didactic)

1. Background
   Didactic _____
   Lab _____
   Peer _____
   ACI _____

2. Equipment
   Didactic _____
   Lab _____
   Peer _____
   ACI _____

3. Verbal encouragement
   Didactic _____
   Lab _____
   Peer _____
   ACI _____

4a. Knee application
   Didactic _____
   Lab _____
   Peer _____
   ACI _____

4b. Ankle application
   Didactic _____
   Lab _____
   Peer _____
   ACI _____

4c. Shoulder application
   Didactic _____
   Lab _____
   Peer _____
   ACI _____

5. Maintenance
   Didactic _____
   Lab _____
   Peer _____
   ACI _____

6. Evaluation
   Didactic _____
   Lab _____
   Peer _____
   ACI _____

7. Recording
   Didactic _____
   Lab _____
   Peer _____
   ACI _____

COMMENTS

_____

_____

_____

_____

_____

_____

_____

_____

Isokinetic Dynamometers

Objective

Develop and demonstrate the skills necessary to use an isokinetic dynamometer to evaluate and develop strength during sport injury rehabilitation.

NATA Athletic Training Educational Competencies embedded in this module: EX-C1, EX-C2, EX-C3, EX-C4, EX-C5, EX-C6, EX-C7, EX-P1, EX-P2, EX-P3, EX-P4, EX-P5, EX-P6, EX-P7, EX-CP1, RM-P1, RM-P2, RM-CP1

Competencies

1. Explain the similarities and differences among isotonic, isometric, and isokinetic resistance.

2. Discuss the similarities and differences among the three principle types of isokinetic dynamometers:
   a. Mechanical
   b. Electrical
   c. Computer generated

3. Demonstrate use of an isokinetic dynamometer for the following:
   a. Measuring knee strength
   b. Measuring shoulder strength
   c. Developing muscular strength, by performing the elements of therapeutic exercise in this list:
   – Set up the equipment.
   – Position the patient.
   – Stabilize the patient during repetitions.
   – Demonstrate proper execution of repetitions (form, timing, control).
   – Explain how and when to adjust the equipment.
   – Demonstrate ways an athlete can cheat on the equipment.
   – Outline safety factors for the athlete and yourself.
   – Demonstrate how to record results.
   – Demonstrate and explain maintenance and simple repair procedures.

Proficiency Demonstration

1. Develop appropriate subject knowledge through coursework (C), verbal conversation (V), quizzes (Q), worksheets (W), or other approved activities (O).

2. Practice and reinforce the skills in clinical skills and laboratory courses.

3. Refine your skills by observing peer teachers and clinical instructors as they perform the skills (preferably on patients), discussing the competencies with peer teachers and clinical instructors, practicing alone and with others, and then demonstrating proficiency to a peer teacher.

4. Demonstrate your proficiency to an ACI.

APPROVED BY
(date and signature, and mode for didactic)

1. Resistance types
   Didactic _____
   Lab _____
   Peer _____
   ACI _____

2. Isokinetic devices
   Didactic _____
   Lab _____
   Peer _____
   ACI _____

3a. Measuring knee strength
   Didactic _____
   Lab _____
   Peer _____
   ACI _____

3b. Measuring shoulder strength
   Didactic _____
   Lab _____
   Peer _____
   ACI _____

3c. Developing muscle strength
   Didactic _____
   Lab _____
   Peer _____
   ACI _____

COMMENTS

_____

_____

_____

Muscular Endurance

Objective

Develop and demonstrate the skills necessary to use therapeutic exercise to improve muscular endurance during sport injury rehabilitation.

NATA Athletic Training Educational Competencies embedded in this module: EX-C1, EX-C2, EX-C3, EX-C4, EX-C5, EX-C6, EX-C7, EX-P1, EX-P2, EX-P3, EX-P4, EX-P5, EX-P6, EX-P7, EX-CP1, RM-P1, RM-P2, RM-CP1

Competencies

1. Discuss the role of improving muscular endurance during sport injury rehabilitation, including when such exercises should be performed during the rehabilitation process.

2. Demonstrate use of the following therapeutic exercises for improving muscular endurance:
   a. Upper body
     – Aquatics
     – Upper-body ergometer (UBE) and stationary bicycle
     – Exercise ball
   b. Lower body
     – Aquatics
     – Stationary bicycle
     – Stair-climber
     – Exercise balls, by performing the elements of therapeutic exercise in this list:
       a. Set up the equipment.
       b. Position the patient.
       c. Stabilize the patient during repetitions.
       d. Demonstrate and instruct proper execution of repetitions (form, timing, control).
       e. Explain how and when to adjust the equipment.
       f. Demonstrate ways an athlete can cheat on the equipment.
       g. Outline safety factors for the athlete and yourself.
       h. Demonstrate how to record the results of the therapeutic exercise session.
       i. Demonstrate and explain maintenance and simple repair procedures for the equipment.

Proficiency Demonstration

1. Develop appropriate subject knowledge through coursework (C), verbal conversation (V), quizzes (Q), worksheets (W), or other approved activities (O).

2. Practice and reinforce the skills in clinical skills and laboratory courses.

3. Refine your skills by observing peer teachers and clinical instructors as they perform the skills (preferably on patients), discussing the competencies with peer teachers and clinical instructors, practicing alone and with others, and then demonstrating proficiency to a peer teacher.

4. Demonstrate your proficiency to an ACI.

APPROVED BY
(date and signature, and mode for didactic)

1. Background
   Didactic _____
   Lab _____
   Peer _____
   ACI _____

2a. Upper body—aquatics
   Didactic _____
   Lab _____
   Peer _____
   ACI _____
   Upper body—UBE and bike
   Didactic _____
   Lab _____
   Peer _____
   ACI _____
   Upper body—exercise ball
   Didactic _____
   Lab _____
   Peer _____
   ACI _____

2b. Lower body—aquatics

Didactic _____

Lab _____

Peer _____

ACI _____

Lower body—bike

Didactic _____

Lab _____

Peer _____

ACI _____

Lower body—stair-climber

Didactic _____

Lab _____

Peer _____

ACI _____

Lower body—exercise ball

Didactic _____

Lab _____

Peer _____

ACI _____

COMMENTS

_____

_____

_____

_____

_____

_____

_____

_____

_____

Aquatic Therapy

Objective

Develop and demonstrate the skills necessary to use pool therapy during sport injury rehabilitation.

NATA Athletic Training Educational Competencies embedded in this module: EX-C1, EX-C2, EX-C3, EX-C4, EX-C5, EX-C6, EX-C7, EX-P1, EX-P2, EX-P3, EX-P4, EX-P5, EX-P6, EX-P7, EX-CP1, RM-P1, RM-P2, RM-CP1

Competencies

1. Define *pool therapy* and explain the following:
   a. Effects
   b. Advantages
   c. Disadvantages
   d. Indications
   e. Contraindications
   f. Precautions

2. Demonstrate and explain the use of a swimming pool for the following:
   a. Increasing joint ROM
   b. Developing muscular endurance
   c. Developing cardiorespiratory endurance
   d. Relieving general muscular soreness
   e. Relieving mental fatigue

3. For each condition, demonstrate and explain the following:
   a. Preapplication procedures
   b. Application procedures
   c. Postapplication procedures

4. Demonstrate proper recording of these treatments on athletic training clinic forms.

Proficiency Demonstration

1. Develop appropriate subject knowledge through coursework (C), verbal conversation (V), quizzes (Q), worksheets (W), or other approved activities (O).

2. Practice and reinforce the skills in clinical skills and laboratory courses.

3. Refine your skills by observing peer teachers and clinical instructors as they perform the skills (preferably on patients), discussing the competencies with peer teachers and clinical instructors, practicing alone and with others, and then demonstrating proficiency to a peer teacher.

4. Demonstrate your proficiency to an ACI.

APPROVED BY
(date and signature, and mode for didactic)

1. Background
   Didactic _____
   Lab _____
   Peer _____
   ACI _____

2a. Increasing joint ROM
   Didactic _____
   Lab _____
   Peer _____
   ACI _____

2b. Developing muscular endurance
   Didactic _____
   Lab _____
   Peer _____
   ACI _____

2c. Developing cardiorespiratory endurance
   Didactic _____
   Lab _____
   Peer _____
   ACI _____

2d. Relieving general muscle soreness
   Didactic _____
   Lab _____
   Peer _____
   ACI _____

2e. Relieving mental fatigue
   Didactic _____
   Lab _____
   Peer _____
   ACI _____

3. Application

Didactic _____

Lab _____

Peer _____

ACI _____

4. Recording

Didactic _____

Lab _____

Peer _____

ACI _____

COMMENTS

_____

_____

_____

_____

_____

Neuromuscular Control and Coordination Exercises

Objective

Develop and demonstrate the skills necessary to use therapeutic exercise to improve neuromuscular control and coordination during sport injury rehabilitation.

NATA Athletic Training Educational Competencies embedded in this module: EX-C1, EX-C2, EX-C3, EX-C4, EX-C5, EX-C6, EX-C7, EX-P1, EX-P2, EX-P3, EX-P4, EX-P5, EX-P6, EX-P7, EX-CP1, RM-P1, RM-P2, RM-CP1

Competencies

1. Discuss the role of improving neuromuscular control and coordination during sport injury rehabilitation, including when such exercises should be performed during the rehabilitation process.

2. Demonstrate use of the following therapeutic exercises for improving neuromuscular control and coordination:

    a. Upper body
- Proprioceptive neuromuscular facilitation (PNF) patterns
- Proprioception board or balance
- Double- and single-arm balancing
- Wobble board or balance apparatus
- Weighted-ball rebounding or toss

    b. Lower body
- PNF patterns
- Rhythmic stabilization apparatus
- Incline board
- Single-leg balancing

    c. Neck
- Stabilization
- Postural correction

    d. Trunk
- Stabilization
- Postural correction, by performing the elements of therapeutic exercise in this list:
  - Set up the equipment, if necessary.
  - Position the patient.
  - Stabilize the patient during repetitions.
  - Demonstrate and instruct proper execution of repetitions (form, timing, control).
  - Explain how and when to adjust the exercise.
  - Demonstrate ways an athlete can cheat while performing the exercise.
  - Outline safety factors for the athlete and yourself.
- Demonstrate how to record the results of the therapeutic exercise session.
- Demonstrate and explain maintenance and simple repair procedures for the equipment.

Proficiency Demonstration

1. Develop appropriate subject knowledge through coursework (C), verbal conversation (V), quizzes (Q), worksheets (W), or other approved activities (O).

2. Practice and reinforce the skills in clinical skills and laboratory courses.

3. Refine your skills by observing peer teachers and clinical instructors as they perform the skills (preferably on patients), discussing the competencies with peer teachers and clinical instructors, practicing alone and with others, and then demonstrating proficiency to a peer teacher.

4. Demonstrate your proficiency to an ACI.

APPROVED BY
(date and signature, and mode for didactic)

1. Background

Didactic _____

Lab _____

Peer _____

ACI _____

2a. Upper body—PNF patterns

Didactic _____

Lab _____

Peer _____

ACI _____

Upper body—proprioception

Didactic _____

Lab _____

Peer _____

ACI _____

Upper body—arm balance

Didactic _____

Lab _____

Peer _____

ACI _____

Upper body—balance apparatus

Didactic _____

Lab _____

Peer _____

ACI _____

Upper body—weighted-ball rebounding or toss

Didactic _____

Lab _____

Peer _____

ACI _____

2b. Lower body—PNF patterns

Didactic _____

Lab _____

Peer _____

ACI _____

Lower body—rhythmic stabilization apparatus

Didactic _____

Lab _____

Peer _____

ACI _____

Lower body—incline board

Didactic _____

Lab _____

Peer _____

ACI _____

Lower body—single-leg balance

Didactic _____

Lab _____

Peer _____

ACI _____

2c. Neck stabilization

Didactic _____

Lab _____

Peer _____

ACI _____

Neck postural correction

Didactic _____

Lab _____

Peer _____

ACI _____

2d. Trunk stabilization

Didactic _____

Lab _____

Peer _____

ACI _____

Trunk postural correction

Didactic _____

Lab _____

Peer _____

ACI _____

COMMENTS

_____

_____

_____

_____

_____

_____

Muscular Speed Exercises

Objective

Develop and demonstrate the skills necessary to use therapeutic exercise to improve muscular speed during sport injury rehabilitation.

NATA Athletic Training Educational Competencies embedded in this module: EX-C1, EX-C2, EX-C3, EX-C4, EX-C5, EX-C6, EX-C7, EX-P1, EX-P2, EX-P3, EX-P4, EX-P5, EX-P6, EX-P7, EX-CP1, RM-P1, RM-P2, RM-CP1

Competencies

1. Discuss the role of improving muscular speed during sport injury rehabilitation, including when such exercises should be performed during the rehabilitation process.

2. Demonstrate use of the following therapeutic exercises for improving muscular speed:
  a. Reaction drills—upper body
  b. Reaction drills—lower body
  c. Sprint work
  d. Fartlek training, by performing the elements of therapeutic exercise in this list:
    – Set up the equipment.
    – Position the patient.
    – Stabilize the patient during repetitions.
    – Demonstrate and instruct proper execution of repetitions (form, timing, control).
    – Explain how and when to adjust the equipment.
    – Demonstrate ways an athlete can cheat on the equipment.
    – Outline safety factors for the athlete and yourself.
    – Demonstrate how to record the results of the therapeutic exercise session.
    – Demonstrate and explain maintenance and simple repair procedures for the equipment.

Proficiency Demonstration

1. Develop appropriate subject knowledge through coursework (C), verbal conversation (V), quizzes (Q), worksheets (W), or other approved activities (O).

2. Practice and reinforce the skills in clinical skills and laboratory courses.

3. Refine your skills by observing peer teachers and clinical instructors as they perform the skills (preferably on patients), discussing the competencies with peer teachers and clinical instructors, practicing alone and with others, and then demonstrating proficiency to a peer teacher.

4. Demonstrate your proficiency to an ACI.

APPROVED BY
(date and signature, and mode for didactic)

1. Background

Didactic _____

Lab _____

Peer _____

ACI _____

2a. Reaction drills—upper body

Didactic _____

Lab _____

Peer _____

ACI _____

2b. Reaction drills—lower body

Didactic _____

Lab _____

Peer _____

ACI _____

2c. Sprint work

Didactic _____

Lab _____

Peer _____

ACI _____

2d. Fartlek training

Didactic _____

Lab _____

Peer _____

ACI _____

COMMENTS

_____

_____

Objective

Develop and demonstrate the skills necessary to use therapeutic exercise to improve agility during sport injury rehabilitation.

NATA Athletic Training Educational Competencies embedded in this module: EX-C1, EX-C2, EX-C3, EX-C4, EX-C5, EX-C6, EX-C7, EX-P1, EX-P2, EX-P3, EX-P4, EX-P5, EX-P6, EX-P7, EX-CP1, RM-P1, RM-P2, RM-CP1

Competencies

1. Discuss the role of improving agility during sport injury rehabilitation, including when such exercises should be performed during the rehabilitation process.

2. Demonstrate use of the following therapeutic exercises for improving agility:

a. Upper body
  – Throwing
  – Catching
b. Lower body
  – Carioca
  – Crossover
  – Figure eight, by performing the elements of therapeutic exercise in this list:
    • Set up the equipment, if necessary.
    • Position the patient.
    • Stabilize the patient during repetitions.
    • Demonstrate and instruct proper execution of repetitions (form, timing, control).
    • Explain how and when to adjust the exercise.
    • Demonstrate ways an athlete can cheat while performing the exercise.
    • Outline safety factors for the athlete and yourself.
    • Demonstrate how to record the results of the therapeutic exercise session.
    • Demonstrate and explain maintenance and simple repair procedures for the equipment.

Proficiency Demonstration

1. Develop appropriate subject knowledge through coursework (C), verbal conversation (V), quizzes (Q), worksheets (W), or other approved activities (O).

2. Practice and reinforce the skills in clinical skills and laboratory courses.

3. Refine your skills by observing peer teachers and clinical instructors as they perform the skills (preferably on patients), discussing the competencies with peer teachers and clinical instructors, practicing alone and with others, and then demonstrating proficiency to a peer teacher.

4. Demonstrate your proficiency to an ACI.

APPROVED BY
(date and signature, and mode for didactic)

1. Background
Didactic _____
Lab _____
Peer _____
ACI _____

2a. Upper body—throwing
Didactic _____
Lab _____
Peer _____
ACI _____

Upper body—catching
Didactic _____
Lab _____
Peer _____
ACI _____

2b. Lower body—carioca
Didactic _____
Lab _____
Peer _____
ACI _____

Lower body—crossover
Didactic _____
Lab _____
Peer _____
ACI _____

Lower body—figure eight

Didactic _____

Lab _____

Peer _____

ACI _____

COMMENTS

_____

_____

_____

Plyometrics

Objective

Develop and demonstrate the skills necessary to use plyometrics during sport injury rehabilitation to improve upper- and lower-extremity muscular power.

NATA Athletic Training Educational Competencies embedded in this module: EX-C1, EX-C2, EX-C3, EX-C4, EX-C5, EX-C6, EX-C7, EX-P1, EX-P2, EX-P3, EX-P4, EX-P5, EX-P6, EX-P7, EX-CP1, RM-P1, RM-P2, RM-CP1

Competencies

1. Define *plyometrics* and briefly explain its role during sport injury rehabilitation, including when it should be used during the rehabilitation process.

2. Discuss preplyometrics considerations.

3. Outline a plyometrics program for improving upper-body muscular power.

4. Demonstrate use of plyometrics by doing the following for each exercise included in competency 3:
- a. Demonstrate and instruct proper execution of repetitions (form, timing, control).
- b. Explain how and when to adjust the exercise.
- c. Demonstrate ways an athlete can cheat when performing the exercise.
- d. Outline safety factors for the athlete and yourself.
- e. Demonstrate how to record the results of the therapeutic exercise session.

5. Outline a plyometrics program for improving lower-body muscular power.

6. Demonstrate use of plyometrics by doing the following for each exercise included in competency 5:
- a. Demonstrate and instruct proper execution of repetitions (form, timing, control).
- b. Explain how and when to adjust the exercise.
- c. Demonstrate ways an athlete can cheat when performing the exercise.
- d. Outline safety factors for the athlete and yourself.
- e. Demonstrate how to record the results of the therapeutic exercise session.

Proficiency Demonstration

1. Develop appropriate subject knowledge through coursework (C), verbal conversation (V), quizzes (Q), worksheets (W), or other approved activities (O).

2. Practice and reinforce the skills in clinical skills and laboratory courses.

3. Refine your skills by observing peer teachers and clinical instructors as they perform the skills (preferably on patients), discussing the competencies with peer teachers and clinical instructors, practicing alone and with others, and then demonstrating proficiency to a peer teacher.

4. Demonstrate your proficiency to an ACI.

APPROVED BY
(date and signature, and mode for didactic)

1. Background
Didactic _____
Lab _____
Peer _____
ACI _____

2. Preplyometrics considerations
Didactic _____
Lab _____
Peer _____
ACI _____

3. Upper-body program
Didactic _____
Lab _____
Peer _____
ACI _____

4. Upper-body exercises
Didactic _____
Lab _____
Peer _____
ACI _____

5. Lower-body program
Didactic _____
Lab _____
Peer _____
ACI _____

6. Lower-body exercises

Didactic _____

Lab _____

Peer _____

ACI _____

COMMENTS

_____

_____

_____

Cardiorespiratory Endurance

Objective

Develop and demonstrate the skills necessary to use therapeutic exercise to improve cardiorespiratory endurance during sport injury rehabilitation.

NATA Athletic Training Educational Competencies embedded in this module: EX-C1, EX-C2, EX-C3, EX-C4, EX-C5, EX-C6, EX-C7, EX-P1, EX-P2, EX-P3, EX-P4, EX-P5, EX-P6, EX-P7, EX-CP1, RM-P1, RM-P2, RM-CP1

Competencies

1. Discuss the role of maintaining and improving cardiorespiratory endurance during sport injury rehabilitation, including when these activities should be performed during the rehabilitation process.

2. Demonstrate use of the following therapeutic exercises for maintaining and improving cardiorespiratory endurance:
- Upper body
    a. UBE
    b. Stationary bicycle
    c. Stair-climber
    d. Aquatics
- Lower body
    e. Bicycle ergometer
    f. Treadmill
    g. Stair-climber
    h. Aquatics
    i. Running on a field, court, or track

    Do so by performing the elements of therapeutic exercise in this list:
- Set up the equipment, if necessary.
- Position the patient.
- Stabilize the patient during repetitions.
- Demonstrate and instruct proper execution of repetitions (form, timing, control).
- Explain how and when to adjust the exercise.
- Demonstrate ways an athlete can cheat while performing the exercise.
- Outline safety factors for the athlete and yourself.
- Demonstrate how to record the results of the therapeutic exercise session.
- Demonstrate and explain maintenance and simple repair procedures for the equipment.

Proficiency Demonstration

1. Develop appropriate subject knowledge through coursework (C), verbal conversation (V), quizzes (Q), worksheets (W), or other approved activities (O).

2. Practice and reinforce the skills in clinical skills and laboratory courses.

3. Refine your skills by observing peer teachers and clinical instructors as they perform the skills (preferably on patients), discussing the competencies with peer teachers and clinical instructors, practicing alone and with others, and then demonstrating proficiency to a peer teacher.

4. Demonstrate your proficiency to an ACI.

APPROVED BY
(date and signature, and mode for didactic)

1. Background

Didactic _____

Lab _____

Peer _____

ACI _____

2a. Upper body—UBE

Didactic _____

Lab _____

Peer _____

ACI _____

2b. Upper body—stationary bicycle

Didactic _____

Lab _____

Peer _____

ACI _____

2c. Upper body—stair-climber

Didactic _____

Lab _____

Peer _____

ACI _____

2d. Upper body—aquatics

Didactic _____

Lab _____

Peer _____

ACI _____

2e. Lower body—bicycle ergometer

Didactic _____

Lab _____

Peer _____

ACI _____

2f. Lower body—treadmill

Didactic _____

Lab _____

Peer _____

ACI _____

2g. Lower body—stair-climber

Didactic _____

Lab _____

Peer _____

ACI _____

2h. Lower body—aquatics

Didactic _____

Lab _____

Peer _____

ACI _____

2i. Lower body—running on a field, court, or track

Didactic _____

Lab _____

Peer _____

ACI _____

COMMENTS

_____

_____

_____

_____

_____

Activity-Specific Skills

Objective

Develop and demonstrate the skills necessary to use therapeutic exercise to improve activity-specific skills during sport injury rehabilitation.

NATA Athletic Training Educational Competencies embedded in this module: EX-C1, EX-C2, EX-C3, EX-C4, EX-C5, EX-C6, EX-C7, EX-P1, EX-P2, EX-P3, EX-P4, EX-P5, EX-P6, EX-P7, EX-CP1, RM-P1, RM-P2, RM-CP1

Competencies

1. Discuss the role of improving activity-specific skills during sport injury rehabilitation, including when these skills should be performed during the rehabilitation process.

2. Demonstrate use of the following therapeutic exercises for improving activity-specific skills:
   a. Running—speed
   b. Running—endurance
   c. Striking
   d. Throwing
   e. Catching
   f. Swimming
   g. Two other sport activities of your choice, by performing the elements of therapeutic exercise in this list:
   – Set up equipment, if necessary.
   – Position the patient.
   – Stabilize the patient during repetitions.
   – Demonstrate and instruct proper execution of repetitions (form, timing, control).
   – Explain how and when to adjust the exercise.
   – Demonstrate ways an athlete can cheat while performing the exercise.
   – Demonstrate how to record the results of the therapeutic exercise session.
   – Demonstrate and explain maintenance and simple repair procedures for the equipment.

Proficiency Demonstration

1. Develop appropriate subject knowledge through coursework (C), verbal conversation (V), quizzes (Q), worksheets (W), or other approved activities (O).

2. Practice and reinforce the skills in clinical skills and laboratory courses.

3. Refine your skills by observing peer teachers and clinical instructors as they perform the skills (preferably on patients), discussing the competencies with peer teachers and clinical instructors, practicing alone and with others, and then demonstrating proficiency to a peer teacher.

4. Demonstrate your proficiency to an ACI.

APPROVED BY
(date and signature, and mode for didactic)

   1. Background
   Didactic _____
   Lab _____
   Peer _____
   ACI _____

   2a. Running—speed
   Didactic _____
   Lab _____
   Peer _____
   ACI _____

   2b. Running—endurance
   Didactic _____
   Lab _____
   Peer _____
   ACI _____

   2c. Striking
   Didactic _____
   Lab _____
   Peer _____
   ACI _____

   2d. Throwing
   Didactic _____
   Lab _____
   Peer _____
   ACI _____

2e. Catching

Didactic _____

Lab _____

Peer _____

ACI _____

2f. Swimming

Didactic _____

Lab _____

Peer _____

ACI _____

2g. Exercise choice 1

Didactic _____

Lab _____

Peer _____

ACI _____

2h. Exercise choice 2

Didactic _____

Lab _____

Peer _____

ACI _____

COMMENTS

_____

_____

_____

_____

_____

Exercise for the Young and Old

Objective

Develop, demonstrate, and implement knowledge of the physiological and psychological impact of exercise activities on patients of all ages and physical status.

NATA Athletic Training Educational Competencies embedded in this module: DI-C2, EX-C4, EX-P1, EX-P3, EX-P4, EX-P5, NU-C1, NU-C2, NU-C6, NU-C7, NU-C18, NU-C18, NU-C19, NU-C20, NU-P3, NU-CP1, RM-C14, TM-CP1

Competencies

1. Describe selection, instruction, and implementation criteria you would consider in prescribing aerobic exercises for patients in the following age ranges:
    a. 5 to 12 years old
    b. 13 to 17 years old
    c. 18 to 25 years old
    d. 26 to 50 years old
    e. 51 years old and older

2. Describe selection, instruction, and implementation criteria you would consider in selecting anaerobic exercises for patients in the age ranges in competency 1.

3. Describe selection, instruction, and implementation criteria you would consider in prescribing stretching exercises for patients in the ranges in competency 1.

4. Describe selection, instruction, and implementation criteria you would consider in prescribing strengthening exercises for patients in the age ranges in competency 1.

5. Describe selection, instruction, and implementation criteria you would consider in recommending nutritional guidelines for patients in the age ranges in competency 1.

6. Describe preventative measures that physically active people should take to avoid injury and illness. Factor in age, stage of development, intensity, frequency, duration, ergonomics, technique, and so on.

7. Outline the risks and benefits of exercise by special population patients.

Proficiency Demonstration

1. Develop appropriate subject knowledge through coursework (C), verbal conversation (V), quizzes (Q), worksheets (W), or other approved activities (O).

2. Practice and reinforce the skills in clinical skills and laboratory courses.

3. Refine your skills by observing peer teachers and clinical instructors as they perform the skills (preferably on patients), discussing the competencies with peer teachers and clinical instructors, practicing alone and with others, and then demonstrating proficiency to a peer teacher.

4. Demonstrate your proficiency to an ACI.

APPROVED BY
(date and signature, and mode for didactic)

1. Aerobic exercises
    Didactic _____
    Lab _____
    Peer _____
    ACI _____

2. Anaerobic exercises
    Didactic _____
    Lab _____
    Peer _____
    ACI _____

3. Stretching exercises
    Didactic _____
    Lab _____
    Peer _____
    ACI _____

4. Strengthening exercises
    Didactic _____
    Lab _____
    Peer _____
    ACI _____

5. Nutritional considerations
    Didactic _____
    Lab _____
    Peer _____
    ACI _____

6. Preventative measures

Didactic _____

Lab _____

Peer _____

ACI _____

7. Exercise risks and benefits

Didactic _____

Lab _____

Peer _____

ACI _____

COMMENTS

_____

_____

_____

_____

_____

O/P Examination 2

Objectives

Demonstrate your mastery of level 1 and 2 skills.

Competencies

Complete the comprehensive O/P examination with a score of at least 85%.

Proficiency Demonstration

Date taken_____

Score_____

Approved by _____

Reexamination (if necessary)

Date taken_____

Score_____

Approved by _____

Comments

_____

_____

_____

_____

_____

_____

_____

Integrating and Polishing Skills

The modules in this section give students the opportunity to integrate numerous skills as they manage specific injuries. Students will be asked to demonstrate their mastery of related anatomy, as well as their understanding of mechanism, assessment, care, treatment, rehabilitation, and prevention of the injury. Continuation of clinical experiences will afford students the opportunity to work with a variety of sports and situations so that they can improve their proficiency in performing psychomotor skills necessary for an entry-level AT. At this stage of a student's development, the ACI should make every effort to give the student opportunities to apply knowledge and manage various aspects of injury response. Conversely, the student should be an active participant in the learning process. The student must be engaged and participative during the clinical experience and look for opportunities to learn and apply skills. Clinical education is a symbiotic relationship, and its effectiveness is the responsibility of both parties.

Students will also be asked to demonstrate proficiency in communication, teaching, administration, supervision, and professional development. Various projects will be expected as a culmination of the athletic training education. The proficiency of the entry-level AT in communication, administration, and presentation skills is important for future employment and advancement. There are 32 modules in seven groups:

- 4 X modules—Directed Clinical Experience (Athletic Training Staff) 260
- 6 T modules—Peer Teaching and Supervision 266
- 6 N modules—Integrated Injury Management 275
- 6 O modules—Health Care Administration 284
- 3 P modules—Psychosocial Interactions 294
- 6 Q modules—Professional Development 301
- 1 O/P module—O/P Examination 3 311

Level 3.1

Directed Clinical Experience (Athletic Training Staff)

Part of developing the foundational behaviors needed for providing appropriate, legal, ethical, and moral medical care during clinical practice involves the ability to integrate the knowledge and skills into a health care plan for an individual or team. This group of modules allows the student to spread their wings a little and become more independent during their clinical experience. During the course of completion, the modules will require the student to begin accepting health care responsibilities that force the integration of various skills to complete tasks or meet expected goals. Completion of these modules will still require the supervision of an ACI or CI, but it is critical that the supervision morphs from hovering into oversight.

Integrated skills involving injury prevention, acute care, recognition or assessment, treatment, and rehabilitation of patients participating on assigned teams will be necessary for proper completion of these modules. The student should be given various health care responsibilities for an individual team that involve, but are not limited to, team travel, packing, supplies or equipment procurement, emergency plan preparation, emergency plan activation, and various other situational professional expectations.

The clinical experiences required in this section are to serve as the final professional preparation of the next generation of athletic trainers. Every effort should be made to allow for actual experiences with real patients to properly prepare the student for the transition to an entry-level health care professional.

Foundational Behaviors of Professional Practice 3

Objective

Discuss how athletic trainers should conduct themselves when acting in a professional capacity, including behavior toward others, such as patients, professional colleagues, coaches and athletic department staff, and the general public.

NATA Athletic Training Educational competencies embedded in this module: None specifically; these behaviors are to be infused throughout every aspect of the educational program.

Competencies

Define and discuss each of the following as they relate to how you should conduct yourself as you practice athletic training. Include in your discussion how your thinking and patient interaction have changed during your level 2 clinical exercises.

- **a.** Primacy of the patient
- **b.** Team approach to practice
- **c.** Legal practice
- **d.** Ethical practice
- **e.** Advancing knowledge
- **f.** Cultural competence
- **g.** Professionalism

Proficiency Demonstration

1. Develop appropriate subject knowledge through coursework (C), verbal conversation (V), quizzes (Q), worksheets (W), or other approved activities (O).

2. Discuss these principles with a peer and an ACI during clinical experience.

APPROVED BY
(date and signature, and mode for didactic)

1a. Patient primacy

Didactic _____

Lab _____

Peer _____

ACI _____

1b. Team approach

Didactic _____

Lab _____

Peer _____

ACI _____

1c. Legal practice

Didactic _____

Lab _____

Peer _____

ACI _____

1d. Ethical practice

Didactic _____

Lab _____

Peer _____

ACI _____

1e. Knowledge advancement

Didactic _____

Lab _____

Peer _____

ACI _____

1f. Cultural competence

Didactic _____

Lab _____

Peer _____

ACI _____

1g. Professionalism

Didactic _____

Lab _____

Peer _____

ACI _____

COMMENTS

_____

_____

_____

_____

_____

Comprehensive Team Experience

Objective

Polish your skills as you serve as the head student for a specific athletic team during its entire sport season.

Competencies

Work with a specific athletic team during its entire sport season (preseason conditioning through off-season conditioning). Among other responsibilities, do the following:

1. Assist with the physical examination of athletes.
2. Assist with evaluating the team's level of conditioning.
3. Inspect the athletic training clinic for compliance with safety and sanitary standards.
4. Be a team leader in a mock removal from the field or court of an athlete with a possible cervical injury.
5. Inventory equipment and supplies.
6. Prepare an equipment and supply purchase request for the next season based on your inventory.
7. Supervise rotating level 1 and level 2 students assigned to your team as directed by the supervising staff athletic trainer for your team.

Proficiency Demonstration

Obtain the signature of an ACI when you have completed this module.

APPROVED BY
(date and signature, and mode for didactic)

ACI _____

COMMENTS

_____

_____

_____

_____

_____

_____

Clinical Capstone Experience

Objective

Expand your horizons and continue to polish your skills.

Competencies

Serve as a student with another institution (a high school, another college, a professional team, or a sports medicine clinic) for at least 6 weeks or for an athletic team at your institution during the entire sport season, including preseason conditioning, regular season, and off-season conditioning. (Note: This must be in addition to and following module X12.)

Proficiency Demonstration

Obtain the signature of an ACI when you have completed this module.

APPROVED BY
(date and signature)

ACI _____

COMMENTS

_____

_____

_____

_____

_____

_____

_____

_____

Athletic Team Travel

Objective

Learn about expectations of athletic trainers, policies, and procedures for athletic team travel.

NATA Athletic Training Educational Competencies embedded in this module: none

Competencies

1. Discuss the moral, ethical, and legal responsibilities of students traveling independently with athletic teams.

2. Demonstrate understanding of expected standards of care while traveling.

3. Discuss the supplies and equipment you would need to take when traveling with an American football team and another team of your choice

4. Prepare, stock, and pack athletic training supplies and equipment for athletic team travel.

5. Discuss chain of command and EAP information for various aspects of the trip (i.e., travel, hotel, meals, competition, leisure).

6. Prepare and compile emergency contact information for use while traveling.

7. Discuss and role-play scenarios relating to your responsibilities (based on past experience of the ACI) in an attempt to stimulate critical thinking and mental preparation.

Proficiency Demonstration

1. Develop appropriate subject knowledge through coursework (C), verbal conversation (V), quizzes (Q), worksheets (W), or other approved activities (O).

2. Practice and reinforce the skills in clinical skills and laboratory courses.

3. Refine your skills by observing peer teachers and clinical instructors as they perform the skills (preferably on patients), discussing the competencies with peer teachers and clinical instructors, practicing alone and with others, and then demonstrating proficiency to a peer teacher.

4. Demonstrate your proficiency to an ACI.

APPROVED BY
(date and signature, and mode for didactic)

1. Responsibilities

Didactic _____

Lab _____

Peer _____

ACI _____

2. Standard of care

Didactic _____

Lab _____

Peer _____

ACI _____

3. Supplies and equipment discussion

Didactic _____

Lab _____

Peer _____

ACI _____

4. Packing supplies and equipment

Didactic _____

Lab _____

Peer _____

ACI _____

5. EAP

Didactic _____

Lab _____

Peer _____

ACI _____

6. Contact information

Didactic _____

Lab _____

Peer _____

ACI _____

7. Scenarios

Didactic _____

Lab _____

Peer _____

ACI _____

COMMENTS

_____

_____

_____

Level 3.2

Peer Teaching and Supervision

Peer teaching and learning should never end. Life-long learning from professional colleagues has professional value that can never be truly measured. The peer teaching and supervision modules in this section continue the practice started earlier in this program. In these modules, level 3 students continue to teach fellow students as they progress through the levels 2 and 3 modules. In addition, students are expected to help their educators write and administer the programs' O/P questions and examinations.

Teaching and Supervising Level 2 Students

Objective

Teach level 2 skills, assess mastery of those skills by level 2 students, and deepen your own understanding and mastery of those skills.

Competencies

1. Peer teach at least four level 2 students and at least 15 level 2 modules. This includes reviewing material with the students, offering suggestions and corrections as they practice the skills, and then assessing their mastery of the skill when appropriate. Students must practice the skills long enough that they become proficient before assessment. Refer often to references and teaching aids.

2. Discuss your peer teaching experience with a faculty AT or clinical instructor.

Proficiency Demonstration

1. Record your peer teaching experiences in the spaces provided:

Name of student	Module	Review date	Assessment date
1.			
2.			
3.			
4.			
5.			
6.			
7.			
8.			
9.			
10.			
11.			
12.			
13.			
14.			
15.			
16.			
17.			
18.			
19.			
20.			
21.			
22.			
23.			
24.			

Name of student	Module	Review date	Assessment date
25. _____	_____	_____	_____
26. _____	_____	_____	_____
27. _____	_____	_____	_____
28. _____	_____	_____	_____
29. _____	_____	_____	_____
30. _____	_____	_____	_____

2. Task completed and discussed (date) _____

Approved by _____

COMMENTS

_____

_____

_____

Administering O/P Examination 1

Objective

Deepen your understanding and mastery of level 1 and 2 skills by examining others.

Competency

Help your program director examine level 2 students by serving as an examiner for at least five different O/P examinations covering level 1 and level 2 modules.

Person examined   **Date**

1. _____   _____
2. _____   _____
3. _____   _____
4. _____   _____
5. _____   _____
6. _____   _____
7. _____   _____
8. _____   _____
9. _____   _____
10. _____   _____
11. _____   _____
12. _____   _____
13. _____   _____
14. _____   _____
15. _____   _____

Proficiency Demonstration

Peer _____

ACI _____

COMMENTS

_____

_____

_____

Teaching and Supervising Level 3 Students

Objective

Teach level 3 skills, assess mastery of those skills by level 3 students, and deepen your own understanding and mastery of those skills.

Competencies

1. Peer teach at least four level 3 students and at least 10 level 3 modules. This includes reviewing material with the students, offering suggestions and corrections as they practice the skills, and then assessing their mastery of the skill when appropriate. Students must practice the skills long enough that they become proficient before assessment. Refer often to references and teaching aids. *Note:* You must complete all modules within a specific block before you can peer teach others working on modules within that block.

2. Discuss your peer teaching experience with a faculty AT or clinical instructor.

Proficiency Demonstration

Name of student	Module	Review date	Approval date
1.			
2.			
3.			
4.			
5.			
6.			
7.			
8.			
9.			
10.			
11.			
12.			
13.			
14.			
15.			
16.			
17.			
18.			
19.			
20.			
21.			
22.			
23.			
24.			

Name of student	Module	Review date	Approval date
5. _____	_____	_____	_____
6. _____	_____	_____	_____
7. _____	_____	_____	_____
8. _____	_____	_____	_____
9. _____	_____	_____	_____
0. _____	_____	_____	_____

Task discussed (date) _____

Approved by _____

COMMENTS

_____

_____

_____

Administering Comprehensive O/P Examination

Objective

Teach level 3 skills, assess mastery of those skills by level 3 students, and deepen your own understanding and mastery of those skills.

Competency

Help your program director examine level 3 student by serving as an examiner for at least five differen O/P examinations covering level 1, 2, and 3 module

Proficiency Demonstration

Serve as examiner.

Person examined	Date
1. _____	_____
2. _____	_____
3. _____	_____
4. _____	_____
5. _____	_____
6. _____	_____
7. _____	_____
8. _____	_____
9. _____	_____
10. _____	_____

Approved by

ACI _____

COMMENTS

_____

_____

_____

Objective

Refine your teaching skills.

Competency

In consultation with your athletic training program director, select a subject and then write an O/P examination question. Follow the format of questions used by your program.

Proficiency Demonstration

Give a copy of the question to your program director.

APPROVED BY

   ACI _____

COMMENTS

_____

_____

_____

Updating Reference Material

Objective

Help update your athletic training clinic reference library and deepen your own understanding and mastery of those skills.

Competency

Search current literature (texts or professional journals) for two new module references. These may be for the same module or for two different modules. Both references must offer specific information to help students master the skills (competencies) of the module.

Proficiency Demonstration

Give a copy of the complete reference, with full bibliographic citation, to your clinical coordinator.

Approved by (date)

_____

COMMENTS

_____

_____

_____

_____

Level 3.3

Integrated Injury Management

Injury management is a complex and integrated process that involves prevention, risk management, and rehabilitation. It is the process of working to eliminate known risks for injury but also responding appropriately if injuries do occur. It is the overall attempt by the AT to minimize risk and maximize recovery from athletic injuries.

A great painting consists of many individual components that may not hold as much value by themselves as when they are incorporated together. The paper, brush, paint, and frame have value, but probably not as much as when they are used together to meet the artist's goals. Injury management can be viewed in the same way. Though performing individual athletic training clinical skills without consideration of the larger picture may be helpful in many situations, a good AT understands that each skill is only a component within the greater goals for the injury management process. Injury management is a broad and involved clinical proficiency that takes time and practice to develop. It is an intricate balance of what, how, where, and when. It is now time to blend these skills together to form a completed picture.

For completion of these modules, students will be asked to work with an ACI in developing and demonstrating their ability to manage specific patient injuries using the clinical skills from the following module groupings: risk management; acute care of injuries and illnesses; taping, wrapping, padding, and bracing; assessment and evaluation; pharmacology and nutrition; therapeutic modalities; and therapeutic exercise. Integration of these individual skills into a well-coordinated effort to prevent or respond to injuries is the goal of this section.

Every effort should be made to allow students the opportunity to manage injuries with actual patients. It is important to sense the nuances, challenges, emotions, and success of such experiences. Students should work closely with their ACI and become intimately involved in the decision-making process with as many patients as possible. ACI supervision should allow for critical thinking and clinical decision making on the part of the student.

Musculoskeletal Assessment and Diagnosis

Objective

Demonstrate the ability to integrate individual musculoskeletal assessment and diagnostic skills and procedures into a thorough evaluation of musculoskeletal injuries.

NATA Athletic Training Educational Competencies embedded in this module: DI-CP1

Competencies

Integrate the knowledge, skills, techniques, and procedures needed for a comprehensive screening evaluation of an acute musculoskeletal injury or illness of the upper extremity, lower extremity, head and face, and spine and torso. These evaluations should occur with actual patients and include all necessary assessment components to reach an accurate diagnosis and recommendations for continued care. Proper documentation and communication procedures are expected.

Proficiency Demonstration

1. Develop appropriate subject knowledge through coursework (C), verbal conversation (V), quizzes (Q), worksheets (W), or other approved activities (O).

2. Practice and reinforce the skills in clinical skills and laboratory courses.

3. Refine your skills by observing peer teachers and clinical instructors as they perform the skills (preferably on patients), discussing the competencies with peer teachers and clinical instructors, practicing alone and with others, and then demonstrating proficiency to a peer teacher.

4. Demonstrate your proficiency to an ACI.

APPROVED BY
(date and signature, and mode for didactic)

1. Upper-extremity assessment

Peer _____

ACI _____

2. Lower-extremity assessment

Peer _____

ACI _____

3. Head and face assessment

Peer _____

ACI _____

4. Spine and torso assessment

Peer _____

ACI _____

COMMENTS

_____

_____

_____

_____

_____

_____

General Medical Assessment and Diagnosis

Objective

Demonstrate the ability to integrate individual general medical assessment and diagnostic skills and procedures into a thorough evaluation of general medical conditions.

NATA Athletic Training Educational Competencies embedded in this module: MC-CP1

Competencies

Integrate the knowledge, skills, techniques, and procedures needed for comprehensive screening or assessment of general medical conditions and illnesses for at least three patients. These evaluations should occur with actual patients and include all necessary assessment components to reach an accurate diagnosis and recommendations for continued care. Proper documentation and communication procedures are expected.

Proficiency Demonstration

1. Develop appropriate subject knowledge through coursework (C), verbal conversation (V), quizzes (Q), worksheets (W), or other approved activities (O).

2. Practice and reinforce the skills in clinical skills and laboratory courses.

3. Refine your skills by observing peer teachers and clinical instructors as they perform the skills (preferably on patients), discussing the competencies with peer teachers and clinical instructors, practicing alone and with others, and then demonstrating proficiency to a peer teacher.

4. Demonstrate your proficiency to an ACI.

APPROVED BY
(date and signature, and mode for didactic)

   1. Assessment 1

      Peer _____

      ACI _____

   2. Assessment 2

      Peer _____

      ACI _____

   3. Assessment 3

      Peer _____

      ACI _____

COMMENTS

_____

_____

_____

_____

_____

_____

_____

Emergency and Acute Care

Objective

Demonstrate the ability to integrate individual emergency and acute care skills and procedures into proper management and care of acute injury and illnesses.

NATA Athletic Training Educational Competencies embedded in this module: AC-CP1

Competencies

Integrate the knowledge, skills, techniques, and procedures needed for appropriate management of an acute injury or illness for at least three patients. Include initial and secondary assessment procedures, wound care, emergency transportation techniques, documentation, and communication when suitable.

Proficiency Demonstration

1. Develop appropriate subject knowledge through coursework (C), verbal conversation (V), quizzes (Q), worksheets (W), or other approved activities (O).

2. Practice and reinforce the skills in clinical skills and laboratory courses.

3. Refine your skills by observing peer teachers and clinical instructors as they perform the skills (preferably on patients), discussing the competencies with peer teachers and clinical instructors, practicing alone and with others, and then demonstrating proficiency to a peer teacher.

4. Demonstrate your proficiency to an ACI.

APPROVED BY
(date and signature, and mode for didactic)

1. Application 1

Peer _____

ACI _____

2. Application 2

Peer _____

ACI _____

3. Application 3

Peer _____

ACI _____

COMMENTS

_____

_____

_____

_____

_____

Rehabilitation Overview

Objective

Demonstrate the ability to design a rehabilitation program that will progress an athlete from injury to full sport participation.

NATA Athletic Training Educational Competencies embedded in this module: EX-C1, EX-C4, EX-C5, EX-C6, EX-C7, EX-C8,TM-C1, TM-C9

Competencies

1. Outline and discuss a rehabilitation program for an injury of your choice. Include the following components and the reasons why each is necessary.
   a. Evaluation of injury
   b. Phases (i.e., components or core goals)
   c. Goal of each phase
   d. Specific tools you would use to achieve the goals of each phase (e.g., therapeutic modalities, therapeutic exercise)
   e. Criteria for progressing from phase to phase
   f. Assessment tools you would use to determine whether your patient met the progression criteria
   g. Return-to-play criteria
   h. Taping, wrapping, or bracing you would use to protect the injury during practice and competition

2. Discuss the roles of other professionals (e.g., physicians, physical therapists, exercise physiologists) in athletic rehabilitation.

3. Observe and assist your clinical instructor in rehabilitating an injured patient.

Proficiency Demonstration

1. Develop appropriate subject knowledge through coursework (C), verbal conversation (V), quizzes (Q), worksheets (W), or other approved activities (O).

2. Refine your knowledge through discussions with peer teachers and clinical instructors.

3. Demonstrate proficiency to a peer teacher and an ACI.

APPROVED BY
(date and signature, and mode for didactic)

1a. Evaluation

Peer _____

ACI _____

1b. Phases

Peer _____

ACI _____

1c. Goals of each phase

Peer _____

ACI _____

1d. Specific tools

Peer _____

ACI _____

1e. Progression criteria

Peer _____

ACI _____

1f. Assessment

Peer _____

ACI _____

1g. Return-to-play criteria

Peer _____

ACI _____

1h. Taping, wrapping, and bracing

Peer _____

ACI _____

2. Role of health care professionals

Peer _____

ACI _____

3. Observing and assisting the complete process

Peer _____

ACI _____

COMMENTS

_____

_____

_____

_____

Rehabilitation Adherence and Motivation Techniques

Objective

Demonstrate the ability to motivate an athlete during a rehabilitation session.

NATA Athletic Training Educational Competencies embedded in this module: EX-P5, PS-C1, PS-C2, PS-C3, PS-C4, PS-CP2

Competencies

1. Discuss the psychological impact of injury and inactivity on physically active patients.

2. Demonstrate use of the following motivational techniques to lessen the negative psychosocial effects of injury and inactivity often seen during rehabilitation:
  a. Verbal motivation
  b. Visualization
  c. Imagery
  d. Desensitization
  e. Goal setting
  f. Relaxation

3. Discuss techniques for increasing patient compliance with rehabilitation.

4. Discuss methods for preparing and testing an injured athlete's psyche for resumption of activity. Include aspects such as motivation and self-confidence.

Proficiency Demonstration

1. Develop appropriate subject knowledge through coursework (C), verbal conversation (V), quizzes (Q), worksheets (W), or other approved activities (O).

2. Refine your knowledge through discussions with peer teachers and clinical instructors.

3. Demonstrate proficiency to a peer teacher and an ACI.

APPROVED BY
(date and signature, and mode for didactic)

1. Psychological impact

Didactic _____

Peer _____

ACI _____

2a. Verbal motivation

Didactic _____

Peer _____

ACI _____

2b. Visualization

Peer _____

ACI _____

2c. Imagery

Peer _____

ACI _____

2d. Desensitization

Peer _____

ACI _____

2e. Goal setting

Peer _____

ACI _____

2f. Relaxation

Peer _____

ACI _____

3. Patient compliance

Peer _____

ACI _____

4. Readiness to resume activity

Peer _____

ACI _____

COMMENTS

_____

_____

_____

_____

Rehabilitation Planning and Supervision

Objective

Demonstrate mastery of rehabilitative equipment, theory, practice, and planning by performing comprehensive rehabilitation of injured patients.

NATA Athletic Training Educational Competencies embedded in this module: AD-P5, AD-P5, EX-P1, EX-P2, EX-P3, EX-P4, EX-P5, EX-P6, EX-P7, EX-CP1, TM-CP1

Competencies

1. Plan and supervise the rehabilitation of four patients with the conditions outlined in the following list. Include the procedures outlined in competency 2. Get approval of your clinical instructor for each phase of the rehabilitation, but the majority of the planning and execution must be done by you.

At least one of the following must be an acute injury and one a postsurgical injury:
   a. Lower-extremity injury
   b. Upper-extremity injury
   c. Trunk injury
   d. Spine injury

2. Interview and physically examine the patient to establish a working diagnosis and baseline before treatment and rehabilitation. Based on the data obtained, do the following:
   a. Determine intervention (therapeutic modality and therapeutic and functional exercise), indications, contraindications, and precautions.
   b. Set medium- and short-range rehabilitative goals.
   c. Research evidence based-data concerning appropriate intervention.
   d. Select appropriate intervention to meet rehabilitative goals.
   e. Inspect equipment to determine that it is operating safely.
   f. Instruct the patient on use and safety measures for rehabilitative exercise equipment.
   g. Provide appropriate psychosocial interventions and motivational techniques throughout the process.
   h. Consult with or refer the patient to other medical and health care professionals as needed.
   i. Monitor the patient during limited practice as appropriate.
   j. Functionally assess progress and recovery throughout the process.
   k. Adjust goals and intervention as indicated by objective progress and psychosocial assessment.
   l. Communicate progress to all interested parties as appropriate (e.g., patient, family, coaches).
   m. Record all intervention, testing data, and progress.
   n. Release the patient to full activity when appropriate

Proficiency Demonstration

Complete steps 2a through 2m for four patients. Consult your texts, notes, and clinical instructors as needed.

APPROVED BY
(date and signature, and mode for didactic)

Patient 1

   Condition _____

   Peer _____

   ACI _____

COMMENTS

_____

_____

_____

Patient 2

   Condition _____

   Peer _____

   ACI _____

COMMENTS

_____

_____

Patient 3

    Condition _____

    Peer _____

    ACI _____

COMMENTS

_____

_____

_____

Patient 4

    Condition _____

    Peer _____

    ACI _____

COMMENTS

_____

_____

_____

Level 3.4

Heath Care Administration

Appropriate words to describe the activities that take place in the AT clinic are *multifaceted, varied,* and *diverse.* Prepractice preparation, prevention programs, practice and competition care, assessment, treatment, communication, patient education, risk management, and rehabilitation of patients can take up much of the AT's time. However, in order for the aforementioned responsibilities to be performed well, certain administrative tasks must also be performed.

Inventory, budget supervision, equipment purchases and maintenance, record keeping, human resources issues, policies and procedure development, communication with stakeholders, facility design, facility management, and insurance coverage are just some of the administrative responsibilities that confront ATs who participate in the management and operation of athletic training clinics. Though these activities may not seem glamorous or rewarding, they are necessary for the operation of the more visible work completed in the clinic.

Examining the administrative tasks of various athletic training clinic settings and the people who work in them is helpful in determining individual preferences in future work settings. The following modules are included to facilitate students' understanding of the diverse administrative responsibilities required of ATs. Immersion in administrative duties occurs immediately upon employment, and there is little time for on-the-job training. Therefore, it is imperative that both the student and clinical instructor seek opportunities during the educational process for supervised involvement in the administrative duties required for effective operation of an athletic training clinic.

Program Policies and Procedures

Objective

Understand basic policies and procedures of health care administration and develop administrative skills.

NATA Athletic Training Educational Competencies embedded in this module: AD-C14, AD-C15, AD-C16, AD-C17, AD-P1, AD-P2, AD-P3,

Competency

1. Demonstrate your understanding of vision and mission statements by discussing the following about each:

    a. Purpose

    b. Important elements

    c. Examples of effective statements

    d. Examples of ineffective statements

    e. How they focus the actions of organizations

    f. How they guide strategic planning

2. Discuss the need for regular evaluation of athletic training services, using tools such as WOTS UP (weaknesses, opportunities, threats, and strengths underlying planning) and SWOT (strengths, weaknesses, opportunities, and threats).

3. Discuss the need for a written policies and procedures manual to govern an athletic training department and individual clinics or other health care facilities.

4. Discuss the relationship between policy and procedure in five procedures selected (by a peer and a clinical instructor) from the policies and procedures manual of your facility. For each one, suggest an additional procedure that would support the policy.

5. In consultation with your supervising AT, choose a section of the policies and procedures manual that needs developed or updated. Revise the section and get it approved by appropriate administrators.

6. Discuss elements of first aid and emergency care policies and procedures such as informed consent, incident reports, and so on.

7. Discuss the following components of an EAP for care of acutely injured or ill patents:

    a. Need for such a plan

    b. EAPs for each venue

    c. Personnel education and rehearsal

    d. Emergency care supplies and equipment appropriate for each venue

    e. Availability of emergency care facilities

    f. Communication with onsite personnel and notification of EMS

    g. Availability, capabilities, and policies of community-based emergency care facilities

    h. Community-based managed care systems

    i. Transportation

    j. Location of exit and evacuation routes

    k. Activity or event coverage

    l. Record keeping

8. Develop a risk management plan that will reduce liability and increase safety. Consider the following in your plan:

    a. Security

    b. Fire

    c. Facility hazards

    d. Electrical safety

    e. Equipment safety

    f. Emergency preparedness

Proficiency Demonstration

1. Develop appropriate subject knowledge through coursework (C), verbal conversation (V), quizzes (Q), worksheets (W), or other approved activities (O).

2. Practice and reinforce the skills in clinical skills and laboratory courses.

3. Refine your skills by observing peer teachers and clinical instructors as they perform the skills (preferably on patients), discussing the competencies with peer teachers and clinical instructors, practicing alone and with others, and then demonstrating proficiency to a peer teacher.

4. Demonstrate your proficiency to an ACI.

APPROVED BY
(date and signature, and mode for didactic)

1. Vision and mission statements

    Didactic _____

    Lab _____

    Peer _____

    ACI _____

2. Evaluation and planning

    Didactic _____

    Lab _____

    Peer _____

    ACI _____

3. Need for written policies and procedures manual

Didactic _____

Lab _____

Peer _____

ACI _____

4. Policy and procedure relationship

Didactic _____

Lab _____

Peer _____

ACI _____

5. Updated policies and procedures manual

Didactic _____

Lab _____

Peer _____

ACI _____

6. First aid and emergency policies and procedures

Didactic _____

Lab _____

Peer _____

ACI _____

7. EAP

Didactic _____

Lab _____

Peer _____

ACI _____

8. Risk management plan

Didactic _____

Lab _____

Peer _____

ACI _____

COMMENTS

_____

_____

_____

_____

_____

Human Resources and Personnel Management

Objective

Develop an understanding of principles, practices, policies, and legal requirements of human resources and personnel management.

NATA Athletic Training Educational Competencies embedded in this module: AD-C4, AD-C5, AD-C6

Competencies

1. Discuss common human resources policy, including the following:
   a. Americans with Disabilities Act (ADA)
   b. Equal Employment Opportunity Commission (EEOC) and the federal laws it is charged to enforce
   c. Affirmative action and the federal laws it is charged to enforce
   d. Fair Labor Standards Act (FLSA)
   e. Family and Medical Leave Act (FMLA), Family Educational Rights and Privacy Act (FERPA)

2. Discuss the following aspects of personnel management:
   a. Recruiting and selecting employees
   b. Employee retention
   c. Policies and procedures manual for employees
   d. Personnel policies section in the departmental policies and procedures manual
   e. Employee performance evaluation
   f. Compliance with federal legislation concerning employment practices, such as the legislation listed in competency 1

3. Discuss similarities and differences in personnel management of ATs versus physicians and other medical and allied health care personnel.

4. Discuss principles of designating physicians and other medical and allied health care personnel as official (but unpaid) personnel for your organization.

5. Discuss briefly the following legal concepts concerning the duties and performance of medical and allied health care personnel:
   a. Scope of practice
   b. Standard of care
   c. Liability
   d. Negligence
   e. Informed consent
   f. Confidentiality

Proficiency Demonstration

1. Develop appropriate subject knowledge through coursework (C), verbal conversation (V), quizzes (Q), worksheets (W), or other approved activities (O).

2. Refine your knowledge through discussions with peer teachers and clinical instructors.

3. Demonstrate proficiency to a peer teacher and an ACI.

APPROVED BY
(date and signature, and mode for didactic)

1. Human resources policy and legislation
   Didactic _____
   Peer _____
   ACI _____

2. Personnel management principles
   Didactic _____
   Peer _____
   ACI _____

3. Management of ATs versus other health care personnel
   Didactic _____
   Peer _____
   ACI _____

4. Volunteer personnel
   Didactic _____
   Peer _____
   ACI _____

5. Legal concepts related to performance
   Didactic _____
   Peer _____
   ACI _____

COMMENTS

_____

_____

_____

Facility Management

Objective

Understand the elements of well-designed athletic training facilities and the management of such facilites.

NATA Athletic Training Educational Competencies embedded in this module: AD-C7, AD-C8, AD-C13, AD-C18, AD-P1

Competencies

1. Discuss the role of the Occupational Safety and Health Administration (OSHA) in the management of health care facilities.

2. Discuss federal and state infection control regulations and guidelines concerning the prevention, exposure, and control of infectious diseases.

3. Discuss accreditation of health care facilities, including the similarities and differences among the following agencies:
    a. Joint Commission
    b. Commission on Accreditation of Rehabilitation Facilities (CARF)
    c. Commission on Accreditation of Athletic Training Education (CAATE)

4. Discuss the roles of the agencies in competency 3 in the preparation of health care professionals and the delivery of health care.

5. Describe architectural design elements that facilitate safe and efficient clinical practice facilities.

6. Discuss how the following risks are managed in the health care facility in which you have obtained most of your clinical education:
    a. Security
    b. Fire
    c. Electrical safety
    d. Equipment safety
    e. Emergency preparedness
    f. Hazardous chemicals
    g. Hazardous materials such as those associated with care involving blood, bodily fluids, and infectious diseases

7. Design an athletic training facility that includes at least the following components:
    a. Floor plan (design that is detailed enough to show where furniture and equipment will be located)
    b. Basic acute care, rehabilitation, and treatment areas
    c. Facility evacuation plan
    d. Risk management concepts such as those in competency 6

Proficiency Demonstration

1. Develop appropriate subject knowledge through coursework (C), verbal conversation (V), quizzes (Q), worksheets (W), or other approved activities (O).

2. Refine your knowledge through discussion with peer teachers and clinical instructors.

3. Demonstrate proficiency to a peer teacher and an ACI.

APPROVED BY
(date and signature, and mode for didactic)

1. Role of OSHA

    Didactic _____

    Peer _____

    ACI _____

2. Federal and state infection control

    Didactic _____

    Peer _____

    ACI _____

3. Health care facility accreditation

    Didactic _____

    Peer _____

    ACI _____

4. Educational role of agencies

    Didactic _____

    Peer _____

    ACI _____

5. Architectural design elements

    Didactic _____

    Peer _____

    ACI _____

6. Risk management

    Didactic _____

    Peer _____

    ACI _____

7. Athletic training facility design

Didactic _____

Peer _____

ACI _____

COMMENTS

_____

_____

_____

Fiscal Management

Objective

Develop the ability to manage the fiscal elements of an athletic training program.

NATA Athletic Training Educational Competencies embedded in this module: AD-C10, AD-C11, AD-C12, AD-P8

Competencies

1. Discuss the following budgeting components:
   a. Operations
   b. Capital expenditures
   c. Expendable or supply expenditures
   d. Inventory (capital and expendable)
   e. Needs assessment
   f. Bidding
   g. Institutional purchasing departments

2. Participate in an inventory of capital and supplies of a health care facility in which you obtained clinical education.

3. Develop a budget, including operations, capital equipment, and expendable supplies, based in part on the inventory you performed for competency 2.

4. Describe the benefits and exclusions of the following health insurance and payment models:
   a. Primary insurance
   b. Secondary insurance
   c. Catastrophic insurance
   d. Health maintenance organization (HMO)
   e. Preferred provider organization (PPO)
   f. Medicare
   g. Fee for service
   h. Cash

5. Describe the concepts and procedures of the insurance policy your institution purchases to cover its athletes.

6. Describe the following and how they relate to third-party insurance reimbursement:
   a. Diagnostic codes (ICD-9-CM)
   b. Procedural coding (CPT)

Proficiency Demonstration

1. Develop appropriate subject knowledge through coursework (C), verbal conversation (V), quizzes (Q), worksheets (W), or other approved activities (O).

2. Refine your knowledge through discussions with peer teachers and clinical instructors.

3. Demonstrate proficiency to a peer teacher and an ACI.

APPROVED BY
(date and signature, and mode for didactic)

1. Budgeting components

   Didactic _____

   Peer _____

   ACI _____

2. Inventory participation

   Didactic _____

   Peer _____

   ACI _____

3. Developing a budget

   Didactic _____

   Peer _____

   ACI _____

4. Health insurance and payment models

   Didactic _____

   Peer _____

   ACI _____

5. Institutional insurance policy

   Didactic _____

   Peer _____

   ACI _____

6. ICD-9-CM and CPT coding

   Didactic _____

   Peer _____

   ACI _____

COMMENTS

_____

_____

_____

Objective

Demonstrate the ability to access information and manage data using current computer hardware and software.

NATA Athletic Training Educational Competencies embedded in this module: AD-C2, AD-C3, AD-C9, AD-P4,

Competencies

1. Describe the following elements of a personal computer and demonstrate the ability to use the latter two.

    a. Central processing unit (CPU)

    b. Internal and external storage

    c. Input devices

2. Demonstrate the ability to use the following types of computer software:

    a. Word processor

    b. File management systems

    c. Spreadsheets

    d. Internet

    e. Communication (e-mail)

    f. Budgeting software

    g. Injury-tracking software

3. Discuss other technological needs of an efficient athletic training practice.

4. Review, discuss the highlights of, and demonstrate that you are applying the concepts of module 32 concerning medical record keeping.

5. Discuss the need for record keeping aside from patient medical records in an efficient athletic training practice.

6. Discuss the advantages of paper and electronic record keeping and demonstrate the ability to use both systems.

Proficiency Demonstration

1. Develop appropriate subject knowledge through coursework (C), verbal conversation (V), quizzes (Q), worksheets (W), or other approved activities (O).

2. Practice and reinforce the skills in clinical skills and laboratory courses.

3. Refine your skills by observing peer teachers and clinical instructors as they perform the skills (preferably on patients), discussing the competencies with peer teachers and clinical instructors, practicing alone

and with others, and then demonstrating proficiency to a peer teacher.

4. Demonstrate your proficiency to an ACI.

APPROVED BY
(date and signature, and mode for didactic)

  1. Computer components

    Didactic _____

    Lab _____

    Peer _____

    ACI _____

 2a. Word processor

    Didactic _____

    Lab _____

    Peer _____

    ACI _____

 2b. File management

    Didactic _____

    Lab _____

    Peer _____

    ACI _____

 2c. Spreadsheets

    Didactic _____

    Lab _____

    Peer _____

    ACI _____

 2d. Internet

    Didactic _____

    Lab _____

    Peer _____

    ACI _____

 2e. Communication

    Didactic _____

    Lab _____

    Peer _____

    ACI _____

2f. Budgeting

Didactic _____

Lab _____

Peer _____

ACI _____

2g. Injury tracking

Didactic _____

Lab _____

Peer _____

ACI _____

3. Other technological needs

Didactic _____

Lab _____

Peer _____

ACI _____

4. Review of module B2

Didactic _____

Lab _____

Peer _____

ACI _____

5. Other records

Didactic _____

Lab _____

Peer _____

ACI _____

6. Paper and electronic records

Didactic _____

Lab _____

Peer _____

ACI _____

COMMENTS

_____

_____

_____

_____

_____

_____

_____

_____

Preparticipation Medical and Physical Examination

Objective

Understand the organization and administration of a team or group preparticipation medical and physical examination.

NATA Athletic Training Educational Competencies embedded in this module: RM-C4, RM-C5, AD-C1

Competencies

1. Discuss the concept of wellness screening in general and athletic preparticipation examinations specifically.

2. Discuss the governing principles and goals of athletic preparticipation examinations.

3. Discuss the following concerning preparticipation examinations:

   a. What rules govern them, and what authority established those rules?

   b. What guidelines or recommendations should be followed, and what authority established them?

   c. What are the legal ramifications of ignoring the rules and guidelines?

   d. What components are required?

4. Discuss the following aspects of organizing and administrating a preparticipation medical and physical examination:

   a. Appropriate medical and musculoskeletal examination tests

   b. Selection and organization of site

   c. Forms used to evaluate and record patients' medical history

   d. Responsibilities of personnel involved in the exam

5. Assist in organizing and administering a preparticipation medical and physical examination at your institution, including performing tasks assigned by your clinical instructor. Practice your part if necessary.

Proficiency Demonstration

1. Develop appropriate subject knowledge through coursework (C), verbal conversation (V), quizzes (Q), worksheets (W), or other approved activities (O).

2. Practice and reinforce the skills in clinical skills and laboratory courses.

3. Refine your skills by observing peer teachers and clinical instructors as they perform the skills (preferably on patients), discussing the competencies with peer teachers and clinical instructors, practicing alone and with others, and then demonstrating proficiency to a peer teacher.

4. Demonstrate your proficiency to an ACI.

APPROVED BY
(date and signature, and mode for didactic)

1. Wellness screening

   Didactic _____

   Lab _____

   Peer _____

   ACI _____

2. Preparticipation exam principles and goals

   Didactic _____

   Peer _____

   ACI _____

3. Preparticipation exam policies

   Didactic _____

   Lab _____

   Peer _____

4. Preparticipation exam organization and administration

   Didactic _____

   Lab _____

   Peer _____

   ACI _____

5. Assisting in a preparticipation exam

   Didactic _____

   Lab _____

   Peer _____

   ACI _____

COMMENTS

_____

_____

Level 3.5

Psychosocial Interactions

This section helps students understand essential psychological and sociological interactions of ATs. These interactions are grouped into the following areas: (1) interactions with patients, athletic department personnel, and other community health care providers; (2) recognizing and dealing with substance abuse by patients; and (3) recognizing and dealing with extreme emotional and mental conditions.

ATs often become close to their patients due to almost daily contact with the patient, the service nature of athletic training, and because the AT's sole efforts are to help the patient perform better, as opposed to coaches, who have to be disciplinarians. As a result, ATs often become confidants and therefore are in a position to counsel patients about psychological and social concerns.

Health Care Communication

Objective

Communicate appropriately with the diverse people and interested parties involved in various health care settings.

NATA Athletic Training Educational Competencies embedded in this module: AD-C20, AD-P5, AD-P6, PD-C17, PS-C8, PS-C9

Competencies

1. Discuss communication theories and techniques related to the following:
- a. Interpersonal communication
- b. Ethnic and cultural sensitivity
- c. Projecting a calm, assuring, and authoritative demeanor when discussing a potentially catastrophic injury
- d. Legal, moral, and ethical responsibilities concerning sharing medical information

2. Discuss differences in how you would communicate with patients (adult, adolescent, and child), patients' family and friends (parents, spouse, siblings, roommates), peers, physicians and other allied health care clinicians, supervisors, coaches, administrators, media, community groups (professional and service clubs, boosters), and insurance carriers.

3. Discuss differences among various forms of communication, such as in person; via telephone, e-mail, and texting; and written.

4. Discuss differences in communicating about prevention, acute care, assessment, treatment, rehabilitation, and management procedures to diverse people, such as those listed in competency 2.

5. Discuss appropriate terminology when communicating with various people, such as those listed in competency 2.

6. Discuss how the personality of the person would alter your communication approach, especially with an overbearing, arrogant, or egotistical person.

7. Demonstrate the ability to communicate as outlined in competencies 1 through 4.

8. Accompany a supervising AT on two occasions when communicating in person the status of injured athletes to a coach or coaching staff.

Proficiency Demonstration

1. Develop appropriate subject knowledge through coursework (C), verbal conversation (V), quizzes (Q), worksheets (W), or other approved activities (O).

2. Refine your knowledge through discussions with peer teachers and clinical instructors.

3. Demonstrate proficiency to a peer teacher and an ACI.

APPROVED BY
(date and signature, and mode for didactic)

1. Communication theories and techniques

Didactic _____

Lab _____

Peer _____

ACI _____

2. Diverse people

Didactic _____

Lab _____

Peer _____

ACI _____

3. Diverse forms

Didactic _____

Lab _____

Peer _____

ACI _____

4. Diverse health care topics

Didactic _____

Lab _____

Peer _____

ACI _____

5. Appropriate terminology

Didactic _____

Lab _____

Peer _____

ACI _____

6. Diverse personality types

Didactic _____

Lab _____

Peer _____

ACI _____

7. Demonstrating communication ability

Didactic _____

Lab _____

Peer _____

ACI _____

8. Communicating with coaches

Didactic _____

Lab _____

Peer _____

ACI _____

COMMENTS

_____

_____

_____

_____

_____

_____

_____

_____

Substance Abuse

Objective

Demonstrate the ability to assist a substance-abusing patient in finding professional help.

NATA Athletic Training Educational Competencies embedded in this module: AC-C27, AC-P2, AC-P3, AC-P4, AD-C22, MC-C17, PH-C10, PH-C11, PH-P1, PS-C11, PS-CP1

Competencies

1. Demonstrate understanding of the sociological, physiological, biological, and psychological factors of substance abuse that do the following:
    a. Predispose a person to substance abuse
    b. Induce continuance of substance abuse
    c. Are barriers to cessation
    d. Affect physical performance
    e. Influence behavior
    f. Are warning signs to the health care professional

2. Discuss common performance-enhancing substances, including why they are used, effects (physiological, short and long-term, adverse), and use patterns.

3. Demonstrate the ability to manage (i.e., assess, provide emergency care, activate EMS, monitor, and refer) a patient suffering from a toxic drug overdose.

4. Simulate intervention with a person who has a substance abuse problem, such as with alcohol, tobacco, stimulants, nutritional supplements, steroids, marijuana, or narcotics, and provide an appropriate referral.

5. Simulate a confidential conversation with a health care professional concerning suspected substance abuse by an athlete.

6. Outline the administrative aspects of a prevention program for substance abuse and banned substances, including informational resources, banned substance lists, screening and testing procedures, violation consequences, and treatment protocols.

7. Prepare a list of community resources to which you can refer athletes for substance abuse counseling.

8. Counsel a patient concerning the effects (desired and adverse) of prescribed and over-the-counter medications commonly used by athletes. Include written educational materials.

Proficiency Demonstration

1. Develop appropriate subject knowledge through coursework (C), verbal conversation (V), quizzes (Q), worksheets (W), or other approved activities (O).

2. Refine your knowledge through discussions with peer teachers and clinical instructors.

3. Demonstrate proficiency to a peer teacher and an ACI.

APPROVED BY
(date and signature, and mode for didactic)

1. Understanding substance abuse
    Didactic _____
    Lab _____
    Peer _____
    ACI _____

2. Performance-enhancing substances
    Didactic _____
    Lab _____
    Peer _____
    ACI _____

3. Management of patient suffering from overdose
    Didactic _____
    Lab _____
    Peer _____
    ACI _____

4. Intervention
    Didactic _____
    Lab _____
    Peer _____
    ACI _____

5. Confidential conversation
    Didactic _____
    Lab _____
    Peer _____
    ACI _____

COMMENTS

6. Substance abuse program

Didactic _____

Lab _____

Peer _____

ACI _____

7. Resources

Didactic _____

Lab _____

Peer _____

ACI _____

8. Counseling patient

Didactic _____

Lab _____

Peer _____

ACI _____

Psychosocial Intervention

Objective

Locate the available community resources to which you can refer patients for psychosocial intervention.

NATA Athletic Training Educational Competencies embedded in this module: PS-C1, PS-C2, PS-C3, PS-C4, PS-C5, PS-C6, PS-C7, PS-C8, PS-C9, PS-C10, PS-C11, PS-C12, PS-C13, PS-C14, PS-C15, PS-CP1, PS-CP2

Competencies

1. Discuss theories relating to personality traits, pain perception, locus of control, religious beliefs, personal values, ethnicity, socioeconomic factors, environment, and cultural influences and how they affect the job responsibilities of an AT.

2. Discuss the benefits of, and techniques for, visual imagery, mental preparation, relaxation techniques, desensitization, stress reduction, and motivational skills in acute care, pain control, treatment, rehabilitation, and performance preparation of injured patients.

3. Comprehend and use various personnel management techniques for successful leadership of employees, colleagues, and patients. Techniques include active listening, effective communication, conflict resolution, motivation, personal power, feedback, and goal setting.

4. Describe signs and symptoms of emotional stress, mental disorders, disordered eating, self-destructive behavior, personal crises, and destructive social conflicts.

5. Discuss components of, as well as the need for, a catastrophic injury or event policy for your workplace.

6. Understand the role of various community-based professionals who specialize in psychosocial intervention.

    a. Describe the roles of and demonstrate proper intervention and referral techniques for various health care specialists.

    b. Describe and demonstrate proper communication and record-keeping procedures following referral to health care specialists.

7. Prepare a list of community resources for psychosocial intervention for your patients. Include in this list the professionals' names, specializations, addresses, and phone numbers.

Proficiency Demonstration

1. Develop appropriate subject knowledge through coursework (C), verbal conversation (V), quizzes (Q), worksheets (W), or other approved activities (O).

2. Refine your knowledge through discussions with peer teachers and clinical instructors.

3. Demonstrate proficiency to a peer teacher and an ACI.

APPROVED BY
(date and signature, and mode for didactic)

    1. Psychosocial theory

        Didactic _____

        Lab _____

        Peer _____

        ACI _____

    2. Psychosocial techniques

        Didactic _____

        Lab _____

        Peer _____

        ACI _____

    3. Personnel management

        Didactic _____

        Lab _____

        Peer _____

        ACI _____

    4. Signs and symptoms

        Didactic _____

        Lab _____

        Peer _____

        ACI _____

    5. Catastrophy planning

        Didactic _____

        Lab _____

        Peer _____

        ACI _____

6. Community-based professionals

Didactic _____

Lab _____

Peer _____

ACI _____

7. List of community resources

Didactic _____

Lab _____

Peer _____

ACI _____

COMMENTS

_____

_____

_____

_____

_____

Level 3.6

Professional Development

Professional development activities are imperative for the growth and advancement of professionals and the professional organizations they represent. Although the definition of *professional development* is broad and encompasses many methods, it is essentially focused on continued improvement in areas such as lifelong learning and skill acquisition, understanding and conducting research, dissemination and sharing of information, knowledge of and involvement in professional organizations, understanding of and commitment to professional roles and responsibilities, awareness about governance and regulations of professional practice, and personal marketing and presentation. These activities are all integral components of professional development and serve a twofold purpose of improving the person and the profession.

Professional development for athletic trainers involves intentional advancement of the profession at both a personal and professional level. On the personal level, athletic trainers must be their own best advocate and critic. Practitioners have a responsibility to themselves, their patients, and their profession to continue developing professional behaviors and skills based on personal and professional strengths and weaknesses.

Personal professional development focuses on the importance of continued improvement in the skills, qualities, and knowledge of individual practitioners.

At the organizational level, professional development is more global. It ideally involves continued awareness and promotion of the unique role that the profession plays in society and health care. Becoming involved at local, state, regional, or national levels in promoting and developing the profession is vital for continued employment opportunities in athletic training and advancement of the profession. Each student should be thankful for the work of ATs who have shaped the current state of the profession and participate in opportunities to advance the profession for others.

In the following modules, students will be asked to examine topics that include professional development methods, requirements, and opportunities related to athletic training. Professional development does not end upon graduation or completion of an educational program. Understanding behaviors, regulations, and expectations regarding professional development is critical for both personal and professional advancement.

Regulation of Athletic Training Practice

Objective

Develop and demonstrate understanding of the governance structures, regulations, policies and impact on the profession of various regulatory bodies, policy-making bodies, and agencies that have oversight of the athletic training profession.

NATA Athletic Training Educational Competencies embedded in this module: AD-C17, PD-C1, PD-P2, PD-C3, PD-C5, PD-C6, PD-C7, PD-C8, PD-P2

Competencies

1. Explain the role of the following and their relationships with each other:
   a. State athletic training practice acts
   b. Registration
   c. Licensure
   d. Certification agencies, including the BOC
   e. NATA
   f. CAATE

2. Discuss the following concerning state practice acts:
   a. Legislative processes for enacting, implementing, and updating practice acts
   b. Rationale for regulations to govern the practice of athletic training
   c. Consequences of violating the regulations

3. Describe the scope of practice (roles and responsibilities associated with the practice of athletic training) as outlined in the NATA Athletic Training Educational Competencies and the BOC's Role Delineation Study.

4. Explain the process and benefits of attaining and maintaining athletic training national certification and state licensure, as well as the consequences of violating the regulatory acts of each.

5. Discuss the following concerning continuing education for ATs:
   a. Purpose
   b. Benefits to individual trainers and the profession
   c. Current requirements
   d. How continuing education unit (CEU) credit is determined
   e. Examples of CEU activities
   f. How to locate CEU activities

6. Name the author of, discuss the purpose of, and differentiate among the following documents (have current copies of the documents available as you complete this competency):
   a. NATA Athletic Training Educational Competencies
   b. NATA Standards of practice
   c. NATA Code of ethics
   d. BOC Role Delineation Study
   e. CAATE Standards for the Accreditation of Entry-Level Athletic Training Education Programs

7. Summarize the current requirements for the professional preparation of an AT.

8. Provide evidence that you have accessed the public and policy-making information of the following governing bodies involved in the guidance and regulation of the athletic training profession by providing copies of their current Web pages (specific to the information, not a home page of the association):
   a. State regulatory board
   b. NATA
   c. BOC
   d. CAATE

9. Summarize the position statements issued by the NATA and discuss how these help define the scope of practice of ATs.

Proficiency Demonstration

1. Develop appropriate subject knowledge through coursework (C), verbal conversation (V), quizzes (Q), worksheets (W), or other approved activities (O).

2. Refine your knowledge through discussions with peer teachers and clinical instructors.

3. Demonstrate proficiency to a peer teacher and an ACI.

APPROVED BY
(date and signature, and mode for didactic)

1. Roles and relationships

   Didactic _____

   Peer _____

   ACI _____

2. State practice acts

   Didactic _____

   Peer _____

   ACI _____

3. Scope of practice

Didactic _____

Peer _____

ACI _____

4. Process and benefits

Didactic _____

Peer _____

ACI _____

5. Continuing education

Didactic _____

Peer _____

ACI _____

6. Essential documents

Didactic _____

Peer _____

ACI _____

7. Professional preparation requirements

Didactic _____

Peer _____

ACI _____

8. Accessing information

Didactic _____

Peer _____

ACI _____

9. Position statements

Didactic _____

Peer _____

ACI _____

COMMENTS

_____

_____

_____

_____

_____

_____

Athletic Training in the Community

Objective

Develop and demonstrate an understanding of the roles of ATs in different venues, how these roles and ATs' scope of practice compares to similar health care professionals, and how an AT can communicate with and promote the procession with various community agencies.

NATA Athletic Training Educational Competencies embedded in this module: AD-C19, AD-C20, AD-21, PD-C9, PD-C10

Competencies

1. Discuss the roles of ATs in the following venues:
   a. High schools
   b. Colleges
   c. Professional sport teams
   d. Industrial sites
   e. Hospitals
   f. Community-based health care facilities
   g. Military

2. Develop a strategy to educate the public concerning roles and responsibilities of ATs working in the venues listed in competency 1.

3. Discuss current issues related to providing health care to patients in the venues listed in competency 1. Pay particular attention to insurance policies and payments, public relations, continuing education, performance expectations, and workplace regulations.

4. Describe the scope of practice (roles) of various community-based medical, paramedical, and other health care professions that care for physically active patients.

5. Describe how the scope of practice of ATs is alike and different from those of other health care professionals discussed in competency 4.

6. Describe communication skills necessary for interacting with the professionals discussed in competency 4. Include in this discussion the protocols for referring patients to these professionals.

7. Develop a strategy for promoting the athletic training profession in the community.

Proficiency Demonstration

1. Develop appropriate subject knowledge through coursework (C), verbal conversation (V), quizzes (Q), worksheets (W), or other approved activities (O).

2. Refine your knowledge through discussions with peer teachers and clinical instructors.

3. Demonstrate proficiency to a peer teacher and an ACI.

APPROVED BY
(date and signature, and mode for didactic)

1. Roles of ATs

   Didactic _____

   Peer _____

   ACI _____

2. Current issues

   Didactic _____

   Peer _____

   ACI _____

3. Strategy to educate public

   Didactic _____

   Peer _____

   ACI _____

4. Scope of practice of others

   Didactic _____

   Peer _____

   ACI _____

5. How the scope of practice ATs is alike and different from others

   Didactic _____

   Peer _____

   ACI _____

6. Communication with other professionals

   Didactic _____

   Peer _____

   ACI _____

7. Strategy to promote athletic training

Didactic _____

Peer _____

ACI _____

COMMENTS

_____

_____

_____

LEVEL 3.6

MODULE Q3

Objective

Develop and demonstrate understanding of the history and operation of the NATA as it applies to the education, regulation, and daily practice of athletic training in various settings.

NATA Athletic Training Educational Competencies embedded in this module: PD-C4, PD-C6, PD-C16

Competencies

1. Draw a hierarchical flowchart outlining the organization of the NATA. Include the names of the 10 individual districts along with the states and provinces that are included in them.

2. Use various sources to obtain information that will answer the following questions about the organization:

    a. Who was the first national secretary of the NATA, and what is that person's current title?

    b. What are three official periodicals of the NATA, and when did each start?

    c. What is the contact information for the NATA national office?

    d. What is the Web address of the NATA and your NATA district?

    e. How many people have been elected president of the NATA?

    f. Who is the current NATA president?

    g. Who is the executive director of the NATA?

    h. Who was the first woman president of the NATA?

    i. Approximately how many people are members of the NATA?

3. Examine the history and time line of the athletic training profession and discuss the events that you feel were most critical to the development of the profession.

4. Briefly discuss the history and development of athletic training education and certification. As part of your discussion, tell when education and certification was formally organized, the NATA entity that was responsible for its guidance, and the present governing body.

5. Discuss the role of the NATA in defining and promoting the athletic training profession and health care in general through educational standards, position stands, and participation in joint task forces with other professional organizations.

Proficiency Demonstration

1. Develop appropriate subject knowledge through coursework (C), verbal conversation (V), quizzes (Q), worksheets (W), or other approved activities (O).

2. Refine your knowledge through discussions with peer teachers and clinical instructors.

3. Demonstrate proficiency to a peer teacher and an ACI.

APPROVED BY
(date and signature, and mode for didactic)

1. Organizational flowchart

    Didactic _____

    Peer _____

    ACI _____

2. NATA facts

    Didactic _____

    Peer _____

    ACI _____

3. History and timeline

    Didactic _____

    Peer _____

    ACI _____

4. Education and certification

    Didactic _____

    Lab _____

    Peer _____

    ACI _____

5. Development of the profession and health care

    Didactic _____

    Peer _____

    ACI _____

COMMENTS

_____

_____

Athletic Training Research

Objective

Demonstrate a basic understanding of the research process and the ability to interpret basic professional literature.

NATA Athletic Training Educational Competencies embedded in this module: PD-C13, PD-C14, PD-P4

Competencies

1. Discuss the components and process of scientific research in athletic training.

2. Discuss similarities and differences between qualitative and quantitative research, including the role and characteristics of statistical analysis for each type.

3. Discuss randomized clinical trials research.

4. Discuss the concept of statistical decision making.

5. Demonstrate the ability to interpret a case study by reading about how case studies should be written. Next, read a specific case study published in the past 5 years in a professional journal. Then discuss the following:

   a. Describe the major sections of a properly written case study and the information found in each section. Did the case study you read follow this procedure?

   b. Describe in general how a case study can help you provide better health care. What specific insights did this case provide you?

   c. Describe potential errors you could make when reading and interpreting a case study. How did you avoid these errors when reading the case study?

   d. What questions about the injury or illness presented in the case study did you think of while or after reading the case study? What strategies can you use to answer those questions?

   e. How have you, or will you, apply the results of this case study to your clinical practice?

6. Demonstrate the ability to interpret a literature review by reading about how literature reviews should be written. Next, read a specific literature review published in the past 5 years in a professional journal. Then discuss the following:

   a. Describe the major sections of a properly written literature review and the informa-

tion found in each section. Did the literature review you read follow this procedure?

   b. Describe in general how a literature review can help you provide better health care. What specific insights did this literature review provide you?

   c. Describe potential errors you could make when reading and interpreting a literature review. How did you avoid these errors when reading this literature review?

   d. What questions about the injury or illness presented in the literature review did you think of while or after reading the literature review? What strategies can you use to answer those questions?

   e. How have you, or will you, apply the results of this literature review to your clinical practice?

7. Demonstrate the ability to interpret a research article by reading about how they should be written. Next, read a specific research article published in the past five years in a professional journal. Then discuss the following:

   a. Describe the major sections of a properly written research article and the information found in each section. Did the article you read follow this procedure?

   b. Describe in general how a research article can help you provide better health care. What specific insights did the one you read provide you?

   c. Describe potential errors you could make when reading and interpreting a research article, including failing to identify and consider assumptions the author made. How did you avoid these errors when reading research articles?

   d. What questions about the injury or illness presented in the article did you think of while, or after, reading the article? What strategies can you use to answer those questions?

   e. How have you, or will you, apply the results of this research article to your clinical practice?

   f. Discuss specific research projects that would expand or strengthen the results of the research article you read.

8. Outline and discuss a research project that will answer a question related to athletic training.

Proficiency Demonstration

1. Develop appropriate subject knowledge through coursework (C), verbal conversation (V), quizzes (Q), worksheets (W), or other approved activities (O).

2. Refine your knowledge through discussions with peer teachers and clinical instructors.

3. Demonstrate proficiency to a peer teacher and an ACI.

APPROVED BY
(date and signature, and mode for didactic)

1. Research process

   Didactic _____

   Peer _____

   ACI _____

2. Qualitative versus quantitative research

   Didactic _____

   Peer _____

   ACI _____

3. Randomized clinical trials

   Didactic _____

   Peer _____

   ACI _____

4. Statistical decision making

   Didactic _____

   Peer _____

   ACI _____

5. Interpreting a case study

   Didactic _____

   Peer _____

   ACI _____

6. Interpreting a literature review

   Didactic _____

   Peer _____

   ACI _____

7. Interpreting a research article

   Didactic _____

   Peer _____

   ACI _____

8. Research project

   Didactic _____

   Peer _____

   ACI _____

COMMENTS

_____

_____

_____

_____

Educational Aids and Professional Presentation

Objective

Demonstrate an awareness of health-related educational aids and the ability to make a professional presentation concerning athletic training.

NATA Athletic Training Educational Competencies embedded in this module: AD-C19, PD-C11, PD-C12, PD-P1, PD-P3

Competencies

1. Discuss the availability and general content of health-related educational aids at or near your campus. Include materials such as audiovisual aids, pamphlets, newsletters, professional journals, Web sites, online databases, workshops, and seminars.

2. Collect and organize information about injury prevention and health care appropriate for the following:

    a. People such as health care professionals, patients, parents and guardians, and coaches and other athletic department personnel

    b. Groups such as athletic teams, parent and teacher organizations, and booster clubs

3. Write an outline for a 10-minute presentation of an athletic training topic to one of the following groups of professional acquaintances. Include potential visual aids in the outline.

    a. Health care professionals

    b. Physicians

    c. Parents

    d. Athletic personnel

    e. General public

    f. Athletes and others involved in physical activity

4. Develop your outline into a computer-based presentation (using a program such as PowerPoint® or Corel Presentations), and make the presentation.

5. Discuss the similarities and differences between workshops, seminars, and clinics. Then outline the principles of planning and organizing such events for the various groups listed in competency 3.

Proficiency Demonstration

1. Develop appropriate subject knowledge through coursework (C), verbal conversation (V), quizzes (Q), worksheets (W), or other approved activities (O).

2. Refine your knowledge through discussions with peer teachers and clinical instructors.

3. Demonstrate proficiency to a peer teacher and an ACI.

APPROVED BY
(date and signature, and mode for didactic)

1. Educational aids

Didactic _____

Peer _____

ACI _____

2. Collecting information

Didactic _____

Peer _____

ACI _____

3. Outline

Didactic _____

Peer _____

ACI _____

4. Presentation

Didactic _____

Peer _____

ACI _____

5. Planning and organizing a meeting

Didactic _____

Peer _____

ACI _____

COMMENTS

_____

_____

_____

_____

_____

_____

Presenting Yourself to the Job Market

Objective

Prepare to sell yourself to a potential employer or graduate school.

NATA Athletic Training Educational Competencies embedded in this module: PD-C15

Competencies

1. Visit your college placement bureau and discuss its services with a counselor.

2. Prepare a résumé that outlines your professional preparation and experiences.

3. Write a letter of intent to apply for a professional position or a graduate degree program.

Proficiency Demonstration

1. Develop appropriate subject knowledge through coursework (C), verbal conversation (V), quizzes (Q), worksheets (W), or other approved activities (O).

2. Refine your knowledge through discussions with peer teachers and clinical instructors.

3. Demonstrate proficiency to a peer teacher and an ACI.

APPROVED BY

(date and signature, and mode for didactic)

1. Placement

    Didactic _____

    Peer _____

    ACI _____

2. Résumé

    Didactic _____

    Peer _____

    ACI _____

3. Letter of intent

    Didactic _____

    ACI _____

COMMENTS

_____

_____

_____

_____

_____

_____

_____

O/P Examination 3

Objectives

Demonstrate your mastery of level 1, 2, and 3 skills.

Competencies

Complete the comprehensive O/P examination with a score of at least 85%.

Proficiency Demonstration

Date taken_____

Score_____

Approved by _____

Reexamination (if necessary)

Date taken_____

Score_____

Approved by _____

Comments

_____

_____

_____

_____

_____

_____

_____

Information for Customizing Modules

Individual institutions may choose not to use some of the modules in this text or add modules of their own. If so, the program director should provide a list of changes to the modules. Following are examples of four customized modules. The lists of records, supplies, equipment, and services are used by various institutions for completing the modules. Your clinical supervisor will probably use a different list; these are given merely for illustration.

Module B2—Injury Record Keeping (page 26)

- Daily treatment log
- Individual treatment sheets
- Injury and insurance record
- Physician referral
- Rehabilitation center referral
- Medical history
- Medical history update
- Physician reports
- Computerized injury and treatment report

Module B3—Athletic Training Supplies (page 28)

- Triple antibiotic ointment, 1 oz (30 ml) tube
- 6 in. (15 cm) double-length elastic bandage
- Tolnaftate 1% ointment
- 2-in.-wide (5-cm-wide) Ultra-Light elastic tape, one case
- Second Skin, one jar
- Pro-Wrap underwrap, one case
- Hydrocortisone 1% cream

- 1/8-in.-wide (.3-cm-wide) Steri-Strips
- Lidocaine hydrochloride solution, one bottle
- Fluori-Methane, one bottle
- Afrin, one bottle

Module B4—Athletic Training Clinic Equipment—Small (page 29)

- BioSkin standard knee skin (closed patella), size large
- Active ankle brace, right ankle
- Knee immobilizer splint with Velcro closures
- Groin strap, size medium
- Vacuum splints (bag)
- Philadelphia cervical collar
- Crutches, 1 pair for an athlete who is 6 ft, 10 in. (208 cm) tall
- Full-length spine board

Module C7—Medical Services (page 40)

- Union hospital emergency room
- Union hospital sports medicine
- Regional hospital emergency room
- Regional hospital outpatient room
- Regional hospital sports medicine
- Dr. Robert Burkle's office
- VitaCare—Honey Creek Mall

Reprint of *Hyposkillia and Critical Thinking* for use with Module A2

Athletic Training Education Journal; 2008;3(Jul-Sep):79-81
©by the National Athletic Trainers' Association, Inc.
www.nataej.org

Hyposkillia & Critical Thinking: What's the Connection?

Kenneth L Knight, Editor
Brigham Young University, Provo, UT

Over the summer I read an essay and a book, which continue to press themselves upon my mind and occupy my thoughts: *How Doctors Think* by Groopman.[1] and *Hyposkillia – Deficiency of Clinical Skills* by Fred[2] both contend that physicians' clinical skills suffer because, in the preparation, they are not purposively taught to think critically.

How Doctors Think is about what goes on in a doctors's mind while treating patients.[2; see forward] The idea for it came to Groopman,[1] a physician-educator, while on rounds with students, interns, and residents. In the process of discussing patients, Groopman was disturbed by the lack of depth of his student's questions and thinking. This glaring deficiency lead him to question "Who teaches doctors to think?" Pondering this question lead to discussions with many colleagues, and eventually to a New York Times best selling book. In reflection of his own time as a medical student, Groopman, realized that only "rarely did attending physicians actually explain the mental steps that lead him to his decisions."[1]

One popular approach to help physicians diagnose problems was clinical decision trees — preset algorithms or clinical guidelines that lead from major symptoms through a series of branching questions and eventually to a diagnosis and treatment plan. These, Groopman argued, are fine for "run of the mill diagnosis and treatment," but inadequate when symptoms or tests are vague, conflicting, or inaccurate. Algorithms have their place, he stated, but they also "discourage physicians from thinking independently and creatively. Instead of expanding a doctor's thinking, they can constrain it."[1]

Similarly, Groopman cautions against rigid reliance on the current rage–evidence-based medicine (basing all treatment decisions strictly on statistically proven data). This rigidity suggests rejection of treatment that is not backed by statistical data. Such an approach "risks having the doctor choose care passively, solely by the numbers. Statistics cannot substitute for the human being before you; statistics embody averages, not individuals."[1]

The 10 chapters of *How Doctors Think* are individual case studies of various difficult cases shared with Groopman[1] by various physicians. Recurring themes in these chapters are that physicians often are too quick to make a diagnosis; they do not consider all the possibilities when framing differential diagnosis.

Fred's[2] essay, and his suggestions for medical educators, was so impressive that I sought permission to reprint it in this issue (see p 82). In it, Fred expressed concern at the increasing numbers of "hyposkilliacs" being graduated from medical schools. Hyposkilliacs, he stated are "physicians who cannot take an adequate medical history, cannot perform a reliable physical examination, cannot critically assess the information they cannot create a sound management plan, have little rea power, and communicate poorly...They learn to order all k tests and procedures but don't always know when to order [tl how to interpret them."[2]

Sound familiar? Comments from many athletic trainers past few years convince me that newly graduated athletic suffer from a similar malady. Recent graduates posses knowledge and skills, but suffer from an inability to app knowledge and skills when dealing with actual patients.

Part of the problem, Fred asserted, is due to mental l caused by habitual reliance on technology, which "p physicians from using the most sophisticated, intricate r they'll ever and always have—the brain."[2] As I pondered hi I asked myself a series of questions: Are athletic training s mentally lazy or is there more to it than that? Are we helpi develop critical thinking skills in order to apply the appropri or treatment in each situation? Can they correctly analy patients' responses to that intervention? If so, how is it hap If not, what can be done about it?

Critical Thinking

A common theme between Groopman's[1] and Fred's[2] w the need for greater critical thinking. This is not just a prot physicians, however. Other health professions also cry ou need to develop critical thinking clinicians as well.[3,4]

Despite a good deal having been written about critical t (just try googling "critical thinking"), and how to develop a complex issue and not easy to teach. While developing thinking is an objective of most institutions of higher learn seem effective in teaching it across the curriculum. It ap have become yet another in a long list of educational buzz Gabennesch[7] argues that what most educators teach is at be: critical thinking and that critical thinking has bec "pedagogical fashion that everyone applauds but few conce very deeply."[7]

There are many definitions of critical thinking, rangi simple statements such as "complex, thoughtful, purposeful of forming judgments using reasons and evidence,"[8] comprehensive consensus statement by the American Philos Association, who stated:

"We understand critical thinking to be purposeful, s regulatory judgment which results in interpretati analysis, evaluation, and inference, as well as explana the evidential, conceptual, methodological, riological, or contextual considerations upon which judgment is based. CT is essential as a tool of iry. As such, CT is a liberating force in education and werful resource in one's personal and civic life. While synonymous with good thinking, CT is a pervasive and rectifying human phenomenon. The ideal critical ker is habitually inquisitive, well-informed, trustful of on, open-minded, flexible, fair minded in evaluation, est in facing personal biases, prudent in making ments, willing to reconsider, clear about issues, rly in complex matters, diligent in seeking relevant rmation, reasonable in the selection of criteria, focused quiry, and persistent in seeking results which are as ise as the subject and the circumstances of inquiry nit. Thus, educating good critical thinkers means king toward this ideal. It combines developing CT s with nurturing those dispositions which consistently l useful insights and which are the basis of a rational democratic society."[9]

ortunately, these definitional statements provide little the specifics of the pedagogical implications or practices to teaching critical thinking skills in medical education. pect of teaching critical thinking has been overwhelming, oughts of two authors (Bacon and Brookings) have guided y attempts to engage students in critical thinking. Sir Bacon's[10] advice to readers was:

ad not to contradict and confute,
to believe and take for granted...
to weigh and consider."[10]

itical thinkers are neither cynical (sarcastic, sneering, ing) nor gullible (receive willingly or without question), r they are skeptical (thoughtful, inquiring).

okings[11] identified two characteristics of critical thinkers. ct as critical thinkers, he said, when they:

Identify and challenge the assumptions underlying their own or another's beliefs and behavior, and

Explore and imagine alternatives to current ways of thinking and acting.

pite the fact that everything we do is based on assumptions, ople fail to acknowledge the assumptions that form the f their perspective. Assumptions, (mine, yours, theirs) are n play; whether recognized or not. They are a part of each unique experiential background and affect how each rocesses, and interprets experiences. The following al account (based on actual data) will serve to illustrate this

nors of a study of stretching methods to increase hamstring y conclude that both methods resulted in increased y, but one of the methods is more effective than the other. of a replication of the study conclude that only one of the significantly increases flexibility. What was the e? The second study included 3 groups, a control group in addition to the two experimental groups. Both the control group and one experimental group increased in flexibility, but there was no difference between the two. The act of measuring flexibility was enough of a stimulus to significantly increase flexibility. The supposed increases in flexibility in the lesser of the two experimental groups was the result of measurement rather than the stretching technique. In the first case the authors' conclusion was faulty because they were based on an unrecognized, and faulty assumption that the mere act of measurement would not affect the outcome. The wisdom in actively seeking out assumptions upon which beliefs are based will bring greater clarity and credence to research findings.

But the value of identifying assumptions goes far beyond clarifying research findings. It should become part of everyday life. Educators should help students develop the habit of digging out assumptions upon which their own and others ideas and beliefs are based.

Brookings'[11] second point, that critical thinking involves looking for alternative explanations or conclusions for any given set of findings, is indeed, the essence of differential diagnosis. The inability to view problems from varying perspectives and to consider all possible solutions is not limited only to physicians who, as Groopman[1] suggests, are too quick to render a diagnosis, but is common to much of our society, in all walks of life. When faced with decisions, most make snap judgments without weighing all the evidence, from all sources, and considering all possible alternatives. Conversely, critical thinkers actively seek out alternative explanations, and in comparison, decide which explanation is most likely.

To a large extent, our educational system does not facilitate critical thinking. Much of our education is founded on the lowest level of thinking–rote memorization. Hence students are constrained by a common experiential background that is devoid of the types of experiences that cultivate critical thinking. Such a system allows for maximum exposure but little time for in-depth explorative exercises. Providing early and frequent experiences in which diagnostic thought processes and strategies are overtly discussed would broaden student experiential backgrounds. Once broadened, a student then processes the next experience based upon greater understanding. Then that experience becomes part of his or her personal experiential background, and so on.

Critical thinking involves "processing information, rather than simply absorbing it: analyzing, synthesizing, interpreting, explaining, evaluating, generalizing, abstracting, illustrating, applying, comparing, recognizing logical fallacies."[7] This is not to say that absorbing information by rote memorization is unimportant, rather students must be provided opportunities and encouraged to go beyond memorization to process the information they absorb. Information has to be absorbed before it can be processed.

The same is true with critical thinking. Absorbing, or acquiring critical thinking skills is, of course, only the first step. Follow-up application and practice is necessary to convert this inert skill set into a viable, performative knowledge. Practitioners must *willingly* apply critical thinking skills in order to fully align declarative classroom critical thinking knowledge with real world situations. Educators can greatly facilitate this alignment by modeling such practices both in the classroom and clinical settings.

Clinical Experience and Critical Thinking

Another suggestion from Fred[2] is particularly important to athletic training education. It is that "much of clinical experience should take place in real-world setting, supervised by experienced, compassionate, common sense, real-world practitioners."[2] Real experiences with real patients guided by seasoned, perceptive instructors would convey deeper understanding than the all too often inert classroom knowledge which students have "absorbed."

Many will say, "we do that; an integral part of AT education is clinical experience." Yes we do, but how effective is it? How much clinical thinking does it involve? Four major impediments to critical thinking during clinical experience are: 1) clinical skills courses substitute for too much of students' clinical experience with patients;[13] 2) clinical experience becomes "work" rather than "education;" where students learn by osmosis, i.e. picking up tips and tricks haphazardly; 3) clinical instructors hover too much over students, inadvertently stifling student's autonomous decisions;[13] 4) many clinical instructors do not engage students in critical thinking about their patients. (See Radtke,[14] Table 1 for suggestions). Let's strive to do better.

In summary, I encourage athletic training educators to adopt four specific strategies to purposefully teach and practice critical thinking skills with their students: 1) develop a habit of being skeptical (being neither cynical nor gullible); 2) identify and acknowledge underlying assumptions; 3) consider any and all alternative explanations for a given set of facts, statistics, or circumstances; and 4) create early, and frequent mentored clinical experiences involving autonomous critical thinking and decisions. The goal must be to bridge the gap of classroom knowledge and practical application and thereby help students become knowledgeable, confident, critical thinking professionals.

References

1. Groopman J. How Doctors Think. Boston: Houghton Millfin Co, 2007

2. Fred HL. Hyposkillia – Deficiency of clinical skills . *Texas Heart Institute Journal*. 2005;32(3):255-257.

3. Facione NC, Facione PA, eds. *Critical Thinking and Clinical Reasoning in the Health Sciences: An International Multidisciplinary Teaching Anthology*. Millbrae, CA: The California Academic Press, 2008

4. Profetto-McGrath J..Critical Thinking and Evidence-Based Practice, *Journal of Professional Nursing*, 2005;21(6):364-371

5. Facione PA. *Critical Thinking: What It Is and Why It Counts 2007 Update*. Millbrae, CA: Insight Assessment. Millbrae, CA: The California Academic Press. 2007 Available @ http://www.insightassessment.com/pdf_files/what&why2006.pdf

6 Paul R, Elder L. *Critical Thinking: Tools for Taking Charge of Your Learning & Your Life Life*, (2nd Ed), Upper Saddle River, NJ: Prentice Hall, 2006

7. Gabennesch H. Critical Thinking, What Is It Good for? (In Fa Is It?). *Skeptical Inquirer*. 2006;30(2):36-41. Availa http://www.csicop.org/si/2006-02/thinking.html

8. Paul R., Critical Thinking. Rohnert Park, CA: Sonom University Center for Critical Thinking and Moral Critique,

9 Facione PA. Critical thinking: A statement of expert consen purposes of educational assessment and instrument. The De Report: Research findings and recommendations prepared f committee on pre-college philosophy. Executive Summary, Delphi Report" Millbrae, CA: *The California Academic Pre* 1990. Available online @ http://www.insightassessment.com/pdf_files/DEXadobe.PD

10. Sir Francis Bacon, English author, courtier, & philosopher 1626). Available @ http://www.quoteworld.org/quotes/859

11. Bookfield SD. *Challenging Adults to Explore Alternative Thinking*. San Francisco: Josey-Bass, 1987

12. Facione PA, Facione NC, Giancarlo CA. The Disposition Critical Thinking: Its Character, Measurement, and Relatic Critical Thinking Skill. *Informal Logic,* 2000;20(1):61-84. A @ http://www.insightassessment.com/pdf_files/J_Infrml_Ppr 00%20-%20Disp%20&%20Skls.PDF [cut and paste URL]

13. Knight KL. Progressive Skill Development and Progressive Experience Responsibility. *Athletic Training Education* 2008;3(Jan-Mar):2-4. Available @ http://www.nataej.org/

14. Radtke S. A Conceptual Framework for Clinical Education in Training. *Athletic Training Education Journal*; 2008;2(Apr- 42. Available @ http://www.nataej.org/

Acknowledgment

Thank you to BYU colleagues Mike Diede and Kevi for being sounding boards, and thus helping clarify these t

O/P Examination

O/P examinations are an integral part of athletic training education. Students must pass one of three exams before advancing from level to level and before taking the Board of Certification (BOC) certification exam. Students will also be required to take portions or adaptations of this exam in various athletic training classes, and these adaptations usually will be part of the class grade.

The comprehensive O/P exam may be administered by both faculty and students. When students administer the exam, a minimum of two, but preferably three, students will administer the exam, each marking the exam sheets independently. Students are welcome to videotape their exam but must provide the equipment to do so. In the case of a dispute, the video can be used as evidence, but the tape must contain the entire exam and will be reviewed completely. Previous experience has demonstrated that students lose more points than they gain when the video is reviewed.

Caution

Students are cautioned about using this material exclusively during preparation for taking an O/P exam. Students should prepare by studying the material presented in class. This material is provided to illustrate form and also to neutralize any advantage people think others might have as a result of having old exams from friends.

Grading Exams

Checks are totaled for each question. On some questions the checks are worth a point each; on others they are a half point each. The net points for each question are added, and the total is divided by the total points possible. The three exams are then averaged. If one of the exams deviates (either higher or lower) from the average of the other two by more than 2.5 times, the deviant score is thrown out and the remaining are averaged.

Instructions to Examiners

1. Ask the examinees if they have any questions. If so, answer them as best as you can. If there is some confusion, write the problem on the cover sheet and proceed. The problem will be investigated later.

2. The senior examiner (the one who has been there the longest) reads the first question. If the examinee needs clarification, a second examiner should read the question. If further clarification is needed, the third examiner should read the question, then the first again, and so on. Do not explain further, and do not use your own words.

3. If a person does not get a part of the question right, write what the person said (or failed to say) on the test booklet.

4. Administer this exam yourself. Don't try to look on other examiners' papers to see if they gave credit on one thing or another. You make the decision. If you need to look up a point in a reference text, do so—you'll learn more that way. But do not copy another's work. Make your own judgment.

5. Bring reference works and notes to the exam. You won't be able to use them while taking the exam, but you should have them while administering the exam.

6. Don't worry about your decisions. All three examiners will not mark every question exactly the same. But if you are consistent, everything will average out in the end.

7. The examinee must perform, not tell you what they would do. Except in cases where the question indicates otherwise, if the person does not

perform during the exam, deduct 5 points from the score for that question.

8. Total the number of points for each question immediately after the examinee finishes it. Write this total on the cover sheet of the test booklet, and add it to the cumulative total. By doing this during the exam, you will not have to take time after the exam is over to total the score.

9. Once the exam is over, pile all three exams together facedown and proceed to the next exam. Do not compare scores with the other examiners.

Instructions to the Examinee

These instructions are to be read by examinee before the exam.

1. The supplies intended for your use are on the table. If you believe you need something that is not here, mention how you would use it, and you will be given credit for doing so.

2. Listen to each question carefully. Questions will be repeated as often as you wish, but no further clarifying information will be given.

3. You must act, demonstrate, and perform—not tell what you would do. Saying "I would . . ." usually will cost you points. During observation, state "I am looking for. . . ."

4. Do not actually use tape adherent, and always use underwrap for taping questions. However, indicate whether you would actually use these materials in an actual situation. (This is the one exception to rule 3.)

5. The subject is not allowed to communicate with you in any way. Often it is imperative that you ask the subject questions, however. Tell what a typical answer would be and act accordingly. During some questions it might be appropriate for you to show what you would do if the subject answered the question in different ways.

6. If you have any questions, ask them before the examination begins.

Sample Question

Following is a sample O/P question. It can be modified to fit institutional philosophy and teaching emphasis and can be used as a template for developing additional questions.

Head and Neck Evaluation

Examine an athlete who is down on the field after tackling an opponent. Focus this evaluation primarily on head and neck injuries. You have 7 min. (Note to examiners: Give performance points only if the tasks were actually done. Saying "I would . . ." does not count.)

1. Checking life-threatening situations (ABCs)
   - Airway
   - Breathing
   - Circulation
   - Consciousness
   - Cervical spine complaints
   - Deal with situation immediately if present
   - Tasks performed

2. History of the injury
   - Where hurt
   - How hit
   - Headache
   - Vision
   - Nausea
   - Tinnitus
   - Dizziness
   - Any other body parts that hurt
   - Tasks performed

3. History of the person
   - Previous head injuries
   - Previous neck injuries

4. Observation
   - Abnormal position of head, neck, extremities
   - Lacerations of scalp, head, or face
   - Fluids from ears, nose, or mouth
   - Tasks performed

5. Palpation
   - For pain or point tenderness
   - For bumps or deformity
   - Scalp and head
   - Cervical spine
   - Mastoid process
   - Extremities
   - Tasks performed

6. Testing structural integrity
   - Pupil reaction (constriction–dilation)
   - Pupil tracking
   - Check dermatomes both sides
     - Three in hand
     - Two in forearm
     - Two in upper arm
     - Rationale for evaluating dermatomes
   - Tasks performed
   - Check myotomes both sides
     - Finger apposition, abduction, adduction
     - Finger flexion and extension

- Wrist flexion and extension
- Elbow flexion and extension
- Shoulder abduction and rotation
- Rationale for evaluating dermatomes
  – Tasks performed

7. Testing functional activity

   – Memory—obvious things, not date
   – Mental confusion—count back by 3, 7
   – Neck rotation (while lying on ground)
   – Neck flexion and extension (on ground)
   – Neck lateral deviation (on ground)
   – Tasks performed

8. Decision and action

   – Spine board and ambulance if cervical spine injury suspected
   – Sit up if OK
   – Check balance, pain
   – Stand up if OK
   – Check balance, pain
   – Remove from field if OK
   – Tasks performed

9. Reevaluation

   – Arms outstretched
   – Finger to nose
   – Romberg test
   – Heel to knee
   – Tandem walk
   – Tasks performed
   – Neck motion
     - Active
     - Passive
     - Resistive
   – Dermatomes
   – Myotomes
   – Concussive signs
   – Tasks performed

10. Recording results

    Give five checks if recording results of various tests is mentioned.

    Total checks _____

    Total points _____

    (38 possible—each check is worth 1/2 point)

NATA Competencies Embedded in Modules

The 2006 NATA Athletic Training Educational Competencies are listed below with the modules in which they are embedded. The competencies are organized and labeled as they are in the in the NATA publication. Following are the 12 content areas, with their abbreviations, listed in the order they appear in the NATA book.

1. **RM** Risk Management and Injury Prevention
2. **PA** Pathology of Injuries and Illnesses
3. **DI** Orthopedic Clinical Evaluation and Diagnosis (Assessment and Evaluation)
4. **MC** Medical Conditions and Diseases (General Medical Conditions and Diseases)
5. **AC** Acute Care of Injury and Illness
6. **TM** Therapeutic Modalities
7. **EX** Conditioning and Rehabilitative Exercise (Therapeutic Exercise)
8. **PH** Pharmacology
9. **PS** Psychosocial Intervention and Referral
10. **NU** Nutritional Aspects of Injuries and Illnesses
11. **AD** Health Care Administration
12. **PD** Professional Development and Responsibility

Educational Competency	Modules In Which the Competency Is Embedded
M-C1	G6, X5-12
M-C2	K6
M-C3	G1
M-C4	G1, O6
M-C5	G1, O6
M-C6	C10, E1, H5, K6
M-C7	C4
M-C8	C11, G2
M-C9	C11, X5-11
M-C10	C11
M-C11	G1, G4, I7

Educational Competency	Modules In Which the Competency Is Embedded
RM-C12	G5
RM-C13	G5, I7, M6, M12,
RM-C14	G5
RM-C15	K2
RM-C16	F6-F9, G2, X5-X10
RM-C17	C6, F1-F2, F4-F9, G2, X5-X9
RM-C18	C8, F1-F9, G2
RM-C19	G3
RM-C20	C11
RM-P1	G4-G6, I7, M1-19, X5-X11
RM-P2	G5, M1-M14, X13

Educational Competency	Modules In Which the Competency Is Embedded
RM-P3	G3, M12
RM-P4	F1-F9, G2
RM-P5	C6, F1-F9, G2, X5-X11
RM-P6	C11
RM-CP1	G2, M2-M14, X5-X11
RM-CP2	G2
RM-CP3	C11
PA-C1	E2, K6
PA-C2	E2, K6
PA-C3	E2
PA-C4	E2, E4
PA-C5	C10, E2
PA-C6	E2, K6
DI-C1	E1, E3
DI-C2	E1, M15
DI-C3	E3
DI-C4	B6, I3
DI-C5	B6, M2, M6, M9
DI-C6	I1, I5, J1-J12
DI-C7	I1, J1-J12
DI-C8	I4, J6, J11- J12
DI-C9	I1, J4, J6, J11-J12
DI-C10	I1, J1-J12
DI-C11	I1, I3, J6
DI-C12	I1, I6, I7, J1-6, J8-J10
DI-C13	I1, J1-J12
DI-C14	C11
DI-C15	I1, I3, J1-J6, J8-J19
DI-C16	B6, J1-J12
DI-C17	B2, I1, J1-J12
DI-P1	I2, I8, J1-J12
DI-P2	I8, J1-J12
DI-P3	I3, I8, J6-J7, J11
DI-P4	I5, I8, J1-J12

Educational Competency	Modules In Which the Competency Is Embedded
DI-P5	G1, I6, I8, J1-J6, J8-J11
DI-P6	I6, I8, J1-J6, J8-J11
DI-P7	I8, J1-J12
DI-P8	I8, J1-J12
DI-P9	I4, I8, J11-J12
DI-P10	I8, J1-J12
DI-CP1	J1-J12, N1, P2
MC-C1	E3, K2, K6,
MC-C2	C12, E3, K2-K6
MC-C3	I2, J7, J12, K2-K6
MC-C4	J12
MC-C5	J12
MC-C6	J12
MC-C7	C12, J7, K3
MC-C8	C12, J7, J3
MC-C9	C12, K3
MC-C10	K4
MC-C11	K4
MC-C12	K4
MC-C13	K2
MC-C14	K5
MC-C15	K1
MC-C16	K1-K5
MC-C17	C13, P2
MC-C18	H4, K6
MC-C19	K1-K4
MC-C20	K2
MC-C21	J12
MC-C22	C11, I2
MC-P1	I1, I2
MC-P2	I1, I2, J7, J12
MC-P3	I1, I2, I5, J7
MC-P4	I2, J7, K2-K5
MC-CP1	I1, I2, J7, N2

Educational Competency	Modules In Which the Competency Is Embedded
C-C1	C1, C4,-C6
C-C2	B3-B4, C5-C6, J12
C-C3	B3-B4, C2, C4-C6
C-C4	B6
C-C5	C1-C2, C4-C5
C-C6	B6, C6, J1-J6, J8-J11
C-C7	I2
C-C8	C5
C-C9	C2, C4-C5
C-C10	C1-C2, C4
C-C11	C1-C2, C4
C-C12	C2,C5
C-C13	C5, C9-C10
C-C14	C5, C9
C-C15	C9, C10
C-C16	C1, C4, D1
C-C17	C1, C8
C-C18	C8, E4
C-C19	J12
C-C20	C1
C-C21	J12
C-C22	C6, J6, J11-J12
C-C23	C6
C-C24	C6
C-C25	C6
C-C26	C6
C-C27	C5, C12-C13, K6, P2
C-C28	C10, K6
C-C29	C11
C-C30	C6, D1, K1
C-C31	C6
C-C32	C6
C-C33	C8
C-P1	C2-C5

Educational Competency	Modules In Which the Competency Is Embedded
AC-P2	C3-C5, C12, K6, P2
AC-P3	C3-C5, C9, C11-C12, K6, P2
AC-P4	C3, C5, C8-C9, C11-C12, J12, K1-K6, P2
AC-CP1	N3
TM-C1	E4, L1, L11, N4
TM-C2	L1, L9-L11
TM-C3	L1, L9-L11, N4
TM-C4	E4, L1
TM-C5	L1, L9-L10
TM-C6	L2-L13
TM-C7	L2-L13
TM-C8	B3-B4, L2-L13
TM-C9	L2-L13
TM-C10	L1
TM-C11	L1
TM-P1	L2-L13
TM-P2	L2-L13
TM-P3	L2-L13
TM-P4	L2-L13
TM-P5	L2-L13
TM-P6	L2-L13
TM-CP1	L2-L11, N6, M15
EX-C1	C9, M1-M14, N4
EX-C2	G6, M1-M14
EX-C3	D1-D2, M1-M14
EX-C4	M1-M15, N4
EX-C5	L10-L13, M1-M15, N4
EX-C6	L10, L12, M1-M14, N4
EX-C7	I6, I7, M1-M14, N4
EX-C8	F1-F9, N4
EX-P1	M1-M15, N6, X14
EX-P2	I6, M1-M14, N6, X15
EX-P3	G6, M2,M4-M7, X16

Educational Competency	Modules In Which the Competency Is Embedded
EX-P4	G6, M1-M15, T2-T3
EX-P5	G6, M1-M15, O/P2, T4
EX-P6	M1-M15, T5
EX-P7	M1-M14, T6
EX-CP1	M1-M14, N6, T7
PH-C1	H2
PH-C2	B6, H1-H2
PH-C3	H1
PH-C4	H2
PH-C5	H2
PH-C6	H2
PH-C7	H1
PH-C8	H1
PH-C9	C13
PH-C10	H4, P2
PH-C11	H5, H4, P2
PH-P1	H1, H3-H4, P2
PH-P2	H3
PH-P3	C13
PS-C1	N5
PS-C2	N5, P3
PS-C3	N5
PS-C4	N5, P3
PS-C5	P3
PS-C6	P3
PS-C7	P2, P3
PS-C8	P1, P3
PS-C9	P1, P3
PS-C10	H4, P3
PS-C11	P2. P3
PS-C12	P3
PS-C13	P3
PS-C14	P3
PS-C15	E4, P5

Educational Competency	Modules In Which the Competency Is Embedded
PS-CP1	P3
PS-CP2	N6
NU-C1	H6, M15
NU-C2	H4, H6, M15
NU-C3	H4, H6
NU-C4	H4
NU-C5	H4- H6
NU-C6	H4, M15
NU-C7	H4, M15
NU-C8	H4
NU-C9	H4
NU-C10	H4, H6, M15
NU-C11	H4, M6, M15
NU-C12	H4, H6, M15
NU-C13	C11, H4
NU-C14	H5
NU-C15	H4
NU-C16	H4
NU-C17	H4
NU-C18	G1, M15
NU-C19	H4, M15
NU-C20	H4, M15
NU-P1	G1
NU-P2	H4
NU-P3	H4, H6, M15
NU-CP1	H4, M15
NU-CP2	H5
AD-C1	O6
AD-C2	B2, O6
AD-C3	B2, O5
AD-C4	O2
AD-C5	O2
AD-C6	O2
AD-C7	C9, C10

Educational Competency	Modules In Which the Competency Is Embedded
AD-C8	O3
AD-C9	O5
AD-C10	O4
AD-C11	O4
AD-C12	B3, B4, O4
AD-C13	O3
AD-C14	O1
AD-C15	B1, C3, O1
AD-C16	C3, O1
AD-C17	B1, C1, O2, Q1
AD-C18	B1, C3, O3
AD-C19	Q2, Q5
AD-C20	C7, Q2
AD-C21	C7, Q2
AD-C22	P2
AD-P1	O3
AD-P2	O1
AD-P3	O1
AD-P4	O5
AD-P5	B2, N6, P1
AD-P6	B2, B6, N6, P1
AD-P7	B2, O5

Educational Competency	Modules In Which the Competency Is Embedded
AD-P8	O4
PD-C1	Q1
PD-C2	Q1
PD-C3	Q1
PD-C4	Q3
PD-C5	Q1
PD-C6	Q1, Q3
PD-C7	Q1
PD-C8	Q1
PD-C9	C7, Q2
PD-C10	Q2
PD-C11	Q5
PD-C12	Q5
PD-C13	Q4
PD-C14	Q4
PD-C15	Q6
PD-C16	Q3
PD-C17	P1
PD-P1	Q5
PD-P2	Q5
PD-P3	Q5
PD-P4	Q4

Master Module Completion File

Name _____

(Write the date of completion after your ACI has signed off on the module.)

Level 1 Introduction to AT Clinical Education

1.1 Directed Clinical Experience (Clinic Orientation and Student Staff)

X1

X2

X3

1.2 Developing Clinical Skills

A1

A2

A3

1.3 Athletic Training Clinic Operations

B1

B2

B3

B4

B5

B6

1.4 Emergency and Acute Care of Injuries and Illnesses

C1

C2

C3

C4

C5

C6

C7

C8

C9

C10

C11

C12

C13

1.5 O/P Examination 1

Level 2   Individual Athletic Training Skills Development

2.1 Directed Clinical Experience (Athletic Training Staff)

X4

X5

X6

X7

X8

X9

X10

X11

X12

2.2 Peer Teaching and Supervision

T1

2.3 Surgical Procedures

D1

D2

2.4 The Body

E1

E2

E3

E4

2.5 Taping, Wrapping, Bracing, and Padding

F1

F2

F3

F4

F5

F6

F7

F8

F9

2.6 Risk Management

G1

G2

G3

G4

G5

G6

2.7 Basic Nutrition, Pharmacology, and Wellness

H1

H2

H3

H4

H5

H6

2.8 General Assessment and Evaluation

I1

I2

I3

I4

I5

I6

I7

I8

2.9 Specific Injury Assessment and Diagnosis

J1

J2

J3

J4

J5

J6

J7

J8

J9

J10

J11

J12

2.10 General Medical Conditions, Disorders, and Diseases

K1

K2

K3

K4

K5

K6

2.11 Therapeutic Modalities

L1

L2

L3

L4

L5

L6

L7

L8

L9

L10

L11

L12

L13

2.12 Therapeutic Exercise

M1

M2

M3

M4

M5

M6

M7

M8

M9

M10

M11

M12

M13

M14

M15

2.13 O/P Examination 2

Level 3 Integrating and Polishing Skills

3.1 Directed Clinical Experience (Athletic Training Staff)

X13

X14

X15

X16

3.2 Peer Teaching and Supervision

T2

T3

T4

T5

T6

T7

3.3 Integrated Injury Management

N1

N2

N3

N4

N5

N6

3.4 Heath Care Administration

O1

O2

O3

O4

O5

O6

3.5 Psychosocial Interactions

P1

P2

P3

3.6 Professional Development

Q1

Q2

Q3

Q4

Q5

Q6

3.7 O/P Examination 3

ABOUT THE AUTHORS

Kenneth L. Knight, PhD, is professor of athletic training at Brigham Young University, past chair of the National Athletic Trainers' Association (NATA) Education Council, former editor in chief of the *Journal of Athletic Training*, and founding editor of the *Athletic Training Education Journal*. He has been involved in athletic training education for over 40 years and practiced athletic training for 25 years at the high school, junior college, and collegiate levels.

Knight has taught more than 2,500 students. He was inducted into the NATA Hall of Fame in 2001, the Utah Athletic Trainers' Association Hall of Fame in 2003, and the Rocky Mountain Athletic Trainers' Association Hall of Fame in 2005. He was also named a Most Distinguished Athletic Trainer in 2000 by the NATA. Knight received the Sayers "Bud" Miller Outstanding Educator Award in 1995 and the Clancy Medal for Outstanding Research in Athletic Training from the NATA in 1995 and 1997.

He also is the author of *Cryotherapy: Theory, Technique and Physiology; Cryotherapy in Sport Injury Management; and Therapeutic Modalities: The Art and Science.*

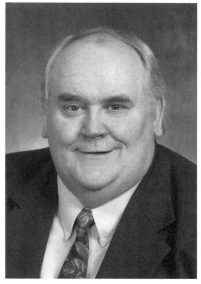

Kenneth L. Knight

Kirk Brumels, PhD, is an associate professor of kinesiology at Hope College in Holland, Michigan. He has been a practicing athletic trainer for more than 20 years, including 11 years in the National Football League with the New England Patriots where he was a member of the 1997 NFL Athletic Training Staff of the Year. Brumels serves as a clinical athletic trainer, didactic and clinical instructor, and director of the athletic training education program at Hope College.

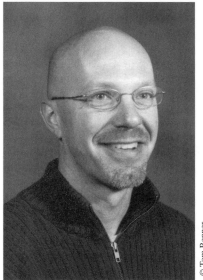

Kirk Brumels

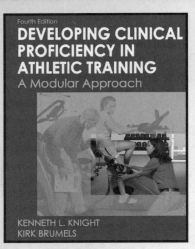
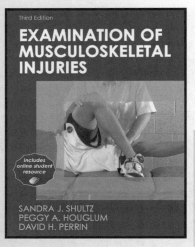
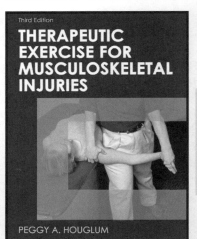
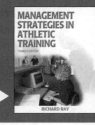
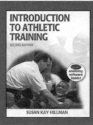